THE
SOCIAL CONSEQUENCES
OF LONG LIFE

THE
SOCIAL CONSEQUENCES
OF LONG LIFE

By

HOLGER R. STUB, Ph.D.

Department of Sociology
Temple University
Philadelphia, Pennsylvania

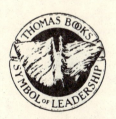

CHARLES C THOMAS • PUBLISHER
Springfield • Illinois • U.S.A.

Published and Distributed Throughout the World by
CHARLES C THOMAS • PUBLISHER
2600 South First Street
Springfield, Illinois, 62717, U.S.A.

© *1982 by* CHARLES C THOMAS • PUBLISHER

ISBN 0-398-04723-5

Library of Congress Catalog Card Number: 82-5775

With THOMAS BOOKS *careful attention is given to all details of manufacturing and design. It is the Publisher's desire to present books that are satisfactory as to their physical qualities and artistic possibilities and appropriate for their particular use.* THOMAS BOOKS *will be true to those laws of quality that assure a good name and good will.*

Printed in the United States of America
CU-R-1

Library of Congress Cataloging in Publication Data

Stub, Holger Richard.
    The social consequences of long life.

    Includes index.
    1. Longevity--Social aspects. 2. Life
expectancy--Social aspects. 3. Old age--Social
aspects. I. Title.
HQ1061.S843   305.2'6   82-5775
ISBN 0-398-04723-5   AACR2

to Elin Holst Stub

PREFACE

DURING the past few years, a considerable amount of material has been written about the apparent increase in life expectancy. With the exception of the effect long life has had on the aging process, relatively little social psychological and sociological analysis has been made of this phenomenon. Though life expectancy increased steadily after the industrial revolution, the most dramatic improvements took place after 1900. The full effect of this important change in the conditions of human life have only begun to be felt throughout the world. It is the relatively slow and often imperceptible change in the chronology of life and death and its consequences that are the subjects of this book.

Twenty years ago, I became interested in the social consequences of high mortality. The idea for this book began to take shape in a lecture that I gave to an undergraduate class in population problems at the University of Minnesota. The conception that the prologation of life at all age levels has an important effect on social life was further developed in several articles. The culmination of this endeavor is presented here.

This book is addressed to students, scholars, other professionals, and laymen who are interested in social change, socialization, the sociology of aging, demography, and social history.

I wish to acknowledge an intellectual debt to some of my teachers: Roy Francis, Arnold M. Rose, and Don Martindale. Other scholars whose work has made an important contribution are Philippe Ariès, Kurt Back, Robert Blauner, Leonard Cain, Jean Fourastié, Peter Laslett, Karl Mannheim, Wilbert E. Moore, Norman Ryder, and Pitirim Sorokin. I further wish to acknowledge my debt to friends and colleagues who have aided by encouragement and critical reading of the manuscript: Jack V. Buerkle, Robert J. Kleiner, Joseph McFalls, and Philip Sagi. Any errors of fact or judgement, of course, are my sole responsibility. The important work of Gloria Basmajian and her staff at the Word Processing

Center and the typing done by Pat Williams and Mary Irene Best was invaluable.

Finally, I owe a great deal to my wife, Elin, who spent many hours in reading and editing my work.

Holger R. Stub
Philadelphia, Pa.

CONTENTS

THE
SOCIAL CONSEQUENCES
OF LONG LIFE

Chapter 1

INTRODUCTION:
A NEW CHRONOLOGY OF LIFE AND DEATH

BIRTH and death form the ultimate boundaries of human existence. Much of the ebb and flow of life is determined by the number and timing of these vital events. An outstanding feature of modern history is the great transformation in the chronology of life. One of the most crucial changes comprising this demographic revolution is that which involves the timing of death and the accompanying increases in length of life. Roughly speaking, this increase in longevity has occurred during the past 250 years, having reached striking proportions during the early decades of the twentieth century.

Mozart was born in 1756, when life expectancy was increasing. His life characterized the ancient human chronology of life and death. Thomlinson writes the following:

> Wolfgang Amadeus Mozart —
> One of seven children, five whom died within six months of birth;
> Father of six children, only two of whom lasted six months;
> Himself a survivor of scarlet fever, small pox, and lesser diseases,
> Only to die at the age of thirty-five and ten months,
> From a cause not diagnosable by the medical knowledge of his time;
> Thus making his life demographically typical of most of man's history. [1]

Though death is ever present and is the concluding act of all men, it makes considerable difference who dies and when it occurs. Over the past two centuries, modern men and women have experienced the conditions of life change, from being short and fraught

3

with uncertainty and misery to being relatively long and substantially free from the fear of imminent death or crippling disease. This change in the chronology is a monumental development in the nature of the human condition.

The aim of this book is to explore some of the social and social psychological consequences of this change in the conditions of human life. It is a basic premise of this work that the change in the timing or pattern of death during the past two centuries is of considerable importance in understanding some of the important features of modern society. However, the available demographic data on the timing of events in the life course of the ordinary person in the societies of the past is scanty and somewhat discomforting to the social scientist. To a considerable degree, we have had to wait for the emergence of a hybrid of demographer-historian-sociologist before any initial analysis of the issue of longevity could be made.[2] An important work in the original planning for this book was that of the French economist-historian, Jean Fourastié.

Jean Fourastié was one of the first modern researchers to clearly perceive the possible social consequences of the dramatic changes in length of life. He derived a *demographic calendar* for males and females in 1730 and 1960. The result is seen in Table 1-I. Life expectancy at birth has tripled, while infant mortality has decreased tenfold. The number of persons per 1000 born alive reaching the marriage age has doubled. Finally, the average European child now loses his first parent through death, at the age of forty instead of fourteen. A new chronology of life and death has developed.

There are at least three salient features of change in the timing of death: (1) the presence of death as a frequent occurrence in social life has greatly diminished; (2) the death rates of the most productive members of society have also been decreased; and (3) this postponement of death has meant a redefinition of both middle and old age, and has delayed the onset of the later by a decade or more.

The rate of increase in longevity that was experienced by most of the birth cohorts (a cohort consists of all those born in a given period, usually one year) living in the industrialized countries after 1700 slowly increased until the late nineteenth century, when the postponement of death reached an accelerating rate. Further improvements appeared after the 1940s with the use of sulpha, penicil-

Table 1-I

The Demographic Calendars for the Average Man and
Woman in Western Europe, 1730-1960

	About 1730		About 1960	
	Males	Females	Males	Females
Life expectancy at birth	25	25	(68)*72	74
Infant mortality per 1,000 born alive	250	230	22	20
Average age at marriage (France)	27	25	26	24
Number of persons per 1,000 born alive reaching above age	425	440	932	952
Average age of average child at the death of the first deceased of his two parents	14 years		40 years	

*Age 72, which appears in the original table, seems to be in error. See Dublin, Louis I.: *Fact-book on Man: From Birth to Death* (2nd edition), New York, MacMillan, 1965, p. 393.

Source: Jean Fourastié, Three comments on the new frontier of mankind, *Diogenes 32*:4, 1960; a technical discussion of the basis for these data is found in : J. Fourastié, Recherches sur le calendrier demographique de l'homme moyen de la vie traditionelle a la vie tertiaire, *Population*, Number 3, 1959, pp. 417-432. Reprinted by permission.

lin, and D.D.T. During this century, the average length of a person's life in the United States has increased by more than 50 percent.

The social changes that have occurred because of the prolongation of life have gone largely unheralded. In contrast, the subject of dying has been vigously studied; aging, gerontology, and geriatrics have taken a prominent place in the scientific arena. In attempting to pursue this investigation of the phenomena of longevity, it was necessary to rely on work done in several seemingly disparate fields of social science and history. The primary data is historical, but of a special variety — that of historical demography. Data on the recent changes in the vital phenomena of birth and death and the broad societal consequences of these differences come from the work of demographers, medieval and social historians, sociologists, and some of the chroniclers of human disaster.

Modern men and women have not only experienced an affluence of goods, but also an addition to their lifetime. Time for living and engaging in social action is the basis of society; the length of time a person has to live and the timing of the major events in the life course are underlying and necessary ingredients in determining the nature of human social life.

Conceptions about the chronology of human life go back to ancient times. The *ages of life* is an early manifestation of our recognition of the rhythm and tempo of human life. The concept of ages of life was a common element in the attempts to understand human biology as far back as the sixth to eighth century A.D. Ariès notes that it originated in the Byzantine Empire and was portrayed graphically in an Arabian fresco in the eighth century.[3] The Athenian poet, Solon, portrayed the ages of life in ten stages of seven years each. It is prominently illustrated in the sonnets of Shakespeare, who depicted seven ages of man.

Though the chroniclers of life have a long history of labeling the definable periods of human life, few people until recent times could realistically hope to live to the last age of life. The prologation of life has meant that for the first time in recorded history the average person will live until he reaches the last age of life. It is well known that a few have always lived much longer than the average; most important however, is the great increase in average age at death. Socially this means that the majority of men and women who have been affected by this revolutionary change will be destined to live on to a life that has been socially uncharted, though well labeled.

Every society develops a general perspective toward life. Such a framework, or point of view, is the result of history and current social and environmental circumstances. For the individual, a given life perspective is the result of one's experience and perception of the predominant features of everyday life. Besides the term *life perspective,* the more general term of *social consciousness* occasionally will be used. This is an abbreviation for the ideas that characterize certain social milieux. It refers to the beliefs, evaluations, conceptions, and images that are generally shared by people of a given social environment. These are reinforced in the consciousness of individuals, by the conviction that they are shared by others in the same group.[4] For example, changes in the frequency and imminence of death dealing disasters will have an impact upon, and result in, changes in the social consciousness of the members of society. Flinn has observed the following: "The outstanding feature of mortality in western Europe in all the centuries before the twentieth has been a great instability. From the highly unstable mortality of, say, the seventeenth century, to the remarkable steadiness of the late twentieth century is a long uneven process of dampening down the fluctuation." That is, "sometimes urban mortality would be highest amongst children, and sometimes amongst adults, whilst life expectancy also varied between men and women."[5]

When the circumstances of everyday life are characterized by the recurrence of famine, disease, accidents, and death, one's perspective is fraught with uncertainty and fear. The greatest concern is then directed at the here and now and an interest in a precise and long range future seems like a frivolous past time. In the same way, the appeal of authority, tradition, ritual, and all that's tried and true is enhanced by an everyday life of uncertainty. Religious, mystical, and magical responses are socially and psychologically functional for such a life perspective, and become an integral part of the social consciousness.

An interesting change has taken place in the attitudes and behaviors associated with the event of death. In traditional societies, men died in the manner of Roland or a Russian peasant. The event was simple and straightforward, and rituals were carried out by the dying person himself, surrounded by family, friends, and neighbors. Children were always included. In fact, it was a public ceremony and the dying man's chamber was open to the public. A point of major importance "is the simplicity with which the rituals of dying were accepted and carried out — in a ceremonial way yes, but with no theatrics, with no great show of emotion."[6]

The following is from Ariès:

> The best analysis of this attitude is found in Alexander Solzhenitsyn's *The Cancer Ward*. Yefrem thought he knew more about death than the old folk. 'The old folk, who never even made it to town, they were scared, while Yefrem rode horses and fired pistols at thirteen. . . . But now . . . he remembered how the old folk used to die back home on the Kama — Russians, Tartars, Votyaks, or whatever they were. They didn't puff

themselves up or fight against it and brag that they weren't going to die —
they took death *calmly* (author's italics). They didn't stall squaring things
away, they prepared themselves quietly and in good time, deciding who
should have the mare, who the foal. . . . And they departed easily, as if
they were just moving into a new house.' [7]

"It could not be better expressed. People had been dying like that
for centuries or millenia. In a world of change the traditional attitude toward death appears inert and static. The old attitude in
which death was both familiar and near, evoking no great fear or
awe, offers too marked a contrast to ours, where death is so frightful
that we dare not utter its name."[8] The change in our view of death,
from the commonplace to the remote and unknown, actually
signifies that a heavy yolk has been lifted from the shoulders of
modern men and women. The psychic consequences of high death
rates among infants, children, youth, and adults have always been
substantial, though seldom studied or discussed. Everyone had too
great a familiarity with death and its required behaviors.

Not only have the roles of mourner, orphan, and widow been
greatly altered, but all of the family roles have been affected.
Mothers and fathers can now allow themselves to become emotionally attached to their small children; they no longer need to defend
themselves psychologically against a child's probable death. No
longer are children familiar with the etiquette and rituals of dying
and death; in fact, most adults are quite unaware of the proper for-
malities until they become middle aged.

The change in the pattern of deaths has had important consequences for the age-old problem of orphanhood. From an early census held in Massachusetts, we learn that from 1830 to 1920, the
number of women who died leaving orphans declined by 87
percent.[9] In 1920, one out of every six children in the United States
lost one or both parents during childhood. By midcentury, the ratio
had dropped to one in twenty. This occurred despite a 37 percent increase in the total number of children.[10] Such a change has
qualitatively altered many aspects of the everyday life of families and
their members.

The steady decline in premature death over the past 200 years
has had considerable effect on the length of marriage. European data
indicates that the average length of marriages in the seventeenth and
eighteenth centuries was fifteen to twenty years. This contrasts with
a projection that French marriages will average approximately

forty-seven years in the 1980s.[11] In essence, the elimination of maternal death has meant that many married women who formerly died in childbirth remain alive. In the past, such deaths allowed single women to marry widowed men. In effect, death gave the marriage market a dynamism that is now provided by divorce.

The general prolongation of life has brought a new set of family roles into being. The postparental stage of family life, when fathers and mothers again live as a couple, came fully into being in about 1900. Prior to that time, death ordinarily claimed one of the parents *before* the last child had left home. These and many other changes in roles and in the quality of family life have resulted from the new chronology of death.

Longevity has had important consequences for education. Two hundred years ago, old age began at fifty, and by then, many of one's age peers were dead. To spend a third to one half of one's anticipated active life in educational preparation would have been virtually unthinkable. An increased life expectancy and the changes wrought by industrialization and increases in wealth provided an important basis for the gradual increase in the time deemed appropriate for education. An example of the changes resulting from longevity and the altered age structure during the past two centuries is illustrated by the average age of the fellows at Kings College, Cambridge University. In 1700, the average age was twenty-five, and in 1937, it was over fifty.[12]

Long life has had a further impact on the education of the young. This is evident in the change in academic evaluation used in schools. Throughout most of the history of formal education, speed of learning has been a major component in the evaluation of ability. When high mortality meant premature death for many, speed in learning was an important and functional requirement. Only that child or youth who possessed extraordinary capabilities had much chance of rising above the traditional lot of peasant or laborer.

The increase in life expectancy and the view of life that has accompanied this change have provided the young with more time to choose an occupation, a partner, and a life-style. The act of choosing alternative courses of action has become a more important component of life than it was when famine and disease made life precarious and short. Being allowed to mature late and, in turn, get needed education without great sacrifice or penalty are new aspects of modern life. The range of possible occupations, approximately 30,000 by official count, demands more time for investigation, experimentation, and planning. The new chronology of life and death helps make this reasonable and possible.

Not only has the prolongation of life made it important to exercise occupational, career, and avocational choices, but status considerations and social mobility have also been affected. The change in the pattern of death has begun to nullify one of the historic status differences, the expected length of life. At the turn of the century, Englishmen in the upper classes had a life expectancy of sixty years. For the lower class level, the figure was thirty years. Much of this difference was due to malnutrition and poor living conditions among the poor.

Long life is a factor in providing the conditions needed for social mobility. Men and women must expect to live well beyond middle age in order to project desires and ambitions beyond those required for a perspective oriented to the present. We must live long enough to allow the fruits of our labor to ripen and bear results in the status struggle. Modern social mobility is partially contingent on education and its system of credentials. Longevity seems to be related to a perspective comprised of future orientation, belief in achievement, and a secular approach to human affairs. Such a perspective is a necessary condition for encouraging and implementing the progressive planning that characterizes the kind of long educational process that has become so important for movement up the status ladder. Moreover, the expectation that one will lead a long and healthy life provides an element of the faith and persistence needed to continue the search for appropriate work and desired status. The added years of living makes first, second, and even third jobs less crucial in determining one's ultimate work career. An uncertain and short life expectancy increases the commitment to early jobs and depresses the willingness to experiment with change in livelihood.

Wolfbein calculated the change in work life that would occur for cohorts of men born in 1900 and 1960. He estimated that 100,000 men born in 1960 would put in approximately one million more man years of work than their counterparts of 1900.[13] This amounts to a 33 percent increase in work time. These data clearly reveal that the changes in the timing of death is closely related to rising levels of living, that is, more time, more work, and more wealth.

The extra time gained from increased length of life has not only increased each person's work contribution to society, but has increased nonwork time as well. Leisure time and retirement have added new dimensions to the lives of modern men and women. In this respect, the most apparent consequence of longevity is that retirement has frequently also meant poverty for the aged. In effect, the added years beyond work life have caught individuals, as well as society, off guard. Inadequate pensions, poor housing, and high priced health services have meant that long life may be a mixed blessing for some. However, certain changes in the economic structure of modern societies may also be positive for the long lived.

The service industries have shown the greatest growth in recent times. Since these industries do not rely on vigorous physical labor, but rather on social and mental skills, the middle-aged and even the "young old" can often function at a fully competitive level with younger workers. This allows for extended years in the labor force. It is true despite the fact that the trend during the past two decades has been towards early retirement. Recent data seem to indicate that this trend is now being reversed.

Long life has made the prospects of having more than one career increasingly possible. In finding the right niche in society, socially and economically, it is now possible to take time for planning and experimentation in the hope of living a more satisfactory life. A personal perspective that views the finding of a satisfactory place in society as a critically important activity may now come to fruition.

The change in chronology of death has had an impact on the aging process of modern industrial society. One of the most obvious consequences is seen in the definition of old age itself. Being defined as old is less and less dependent on chronological age and is increasingly based on one's performance of the social roles associated with a full and active life.

With the new categories of old, it has also become apparent that a successful old age rests on socialization, or learning how to adapt to the aging process at earlier periods in the life course. This has made middle age important as the precursor to old age; success at the earlier period contributes to success later. With the general prolongation of life, middle age has also been lengthened, particularly by the social definition of old age. Old age began earlier among our forefathers because of the rapid depletion of a person's age peers. At fifty-five, men like Henry VIII felt and acted old. Such attitudes resulted from an awareness that one was exceptional if fate kept you alive into the late fiftys or early sixtys.

Long life cannot be credited with positive effects at all stages in the life course. For example, the lengthening of middle age may have contributed to some of the phenomena labeled as "middle-aged malaise," "chaos in middle age," or "middle age depression." The lengthening of middle age and the prospect of old age have forced a certain amount of contemplation and introspection regarding one's past and the prospects for the future. For those who find themselves in middle age with jobs, life-styles, or circumstances that are unsatisfactory, discontent and depression are not unusual. Some can perceive that there yet may be time to make changes and accordingly plan second careers or other changes in life-style.

No society existing before the twentieth century has had the prospect of retirement from work as the normal expectation. This means that the problems that have arisen in coping with this great change have never been faced by human beings before; no prior models of behavior exist. The question of retirement is closely associated with that of leisure. For some, retirement is enforced leisure and, as such, unpleasant. For others, it is a time to increase old pleasures, try new things, and meet new challenges.

The relationship between leisure and long life may have become very important. Throughout the history of the United States (and in much of Europe), leisure has been frequently defined as a time for the re-creation of mind and body so that one can pursue work more effectively. With retirement becoming expected and commonplace, the leisure time associated with it cannot be viewed primarily as recreation for later work. If the leisure associated with retirement is to be socially justified and appropriate, it must have value in its own right. Such a change in the conception of leisure has begun to occur. The turmoil of the 1960s with the questioning of traditional norms and values and the search for alternative life-styles may have contributed to our changing attitude toward leisure. There can be little doubt that the presence of millions of elderly living in leisure has also stimulated a redefinition of leisure.

Long life inevitably means a confrontation with physical decline and susceptibility to degenerative diseases. The realization that we will probably live as "old old" or "frail" members of society has pushed a new dimension of life upon us. It has had a direct impact on such matters as health maintenance through diet, exercise, and preventative medicine. A massive investment of both time and money is being made by the middle-aged and the young old to more effectively meet the anticipated physical and mental problems of old age.

The medical service system is strained to its limits in meeting immediate demands for geriatric care, and this will increase in the future. Long life means that an ample portion of the national product must go for the care of the elderly. New areas of knowledge are emerging, and gerontology is coming into its own. The medical specialty of geriatrics is gaining full recognition. Human genetics is being explored for the possible genetic connections between old age disabilities and the susceptibility to degenerative diseases. We now survive a long list of infectious diseases remaining alive only to fall victim to a whole new set of ills, including losses in our sensory and motor capacities.

The consequences of longevity are occurring in all aspects of human society. Not only does more time to live affect personal lives, but it also influences many large-scale societal aspects of life. The postponement of death all along the life course has meant that more of the persons born at the same time (they comprise a birth cohort) will remain alive and together as a generational force for a longer period of time. During that period of time, each of the cohorts in the early and middle years will die much more slowly than in the past. The change in the timing of death keeps generations intact much longer. This means that each generation may have a greater impact on the history of a period than if they had died more rapidly as in the past. The potential increase in historic impact is due, partly, to the greater number of people remaining alive, and to the fact that social relationships will be more extensive and intricate. This extension and intricacy results from the increased time that the cohorts of a generation share as part of the social fabric of society. At any given point in time, a wide range of cohorts are more completely represented in the social order. Because more cohorts are alive at the same time and contain a larger proportion of their original members, it gives a society greater heterogeneity. This is a result of the increased range of differences between the youngest and the oldest adults and the increased number of aged. The coexistence of numerous birth cohorts across a wide age span reinforces the awareness of social differences and may, in turn, stimulate a diversity of life-styles.

Diversity, a prominent feature of modern society, tends to lead to an increased emphasis on individuality. Long life provides greater scope, and it enhances freedom of choice for the individual, as well as reinforcing the importance of individual and social responsibility. As individuality has increased, its consequences have become more apparent. Movements away from individuality toward collectivization have emerged — a recent example is seen in communal living.

A note about terminology should be incorporated at this point. Throughout this book, terms such as *longevity, extension of life, prolongation of life, life expectancy, average length of life, median age at death,* and *lifespan* will be used. Though all of these terms refer roughly to similar phenomena, some are defined in general impressionistic ways, while others have rather explicit and precise meanings. Longevity, extension of life, and prolongation of life are general terms and will be used to refer to the fact that life expectancies have increased. Expectation of life is expressed as a precise figure. It is determined by taking the total number of years lived by a group, and dividing this number by the total number of people in the group. The median age at death is the age achieved by half of the population in question. The two statistics can vary greatly. For example, a high infant and maternal mortality rate will have a great effect on the life expectancy, whereas its consequences for the median life expectancy (the age at which half the population has died) may be negligible, providing those who survive infancy are not decimated too quickly by other fatal disasters. Lifespan is a term used to indicate the general maximum length of life of human beings. It is believed that the human lifespan has been about 100 years ever since recorded history.[14] The changes in mortality have resulted in larger numbers of people surviving toward this limit.

Life expectancy is now capable of being determined with considerable precision and specificity through the use of life tables. Such tables represent calculations that reveal the probable number of years of life remaining for a hypothetical cohort of persons at each age at a given point in time. These life expectancies are age specific and form the basis for analyzing demographic problems.

Average length of life usually refers to the life expectancy at birth of a whole society in a specific year or time period. Historians and demographers have attempted to determine the average length of life at various times in the past. The following figures have been calculated:[15]

Early Iron and Bronze age, Greece	18 years
Rome, about 2,000 years ago	22 years
Middle ages, England	33 years
Breslau, 1687-1691	34 years
England and Wales, 1838-54	41 years
Before 1789, Massachusetts & New Hampshire	36 years
United States, 1900-1902	49 years
United States, 1946	67 years
United States, 1978	73 years

This data illustrate the important difference between lifespan and average lengths of life. While lifespan has remained quite constant, average length of life varies widely.

Although some of the more technical aspects and specific terminology of this study will be used from time to time, most of the discussion will involve an attempt to explore the broad social consequences of the great change in life expectancies between 1750 and 1980. Life has lengthened to such a degree that it seems to have had revolutionary consequences.

The following chapters will explore the history and some of the social consequences of the new chronology of life. The fact that these changes have taken place over two and a half centuries does not detract from their importance.

REFERENCES AND NOTES

1. Thomlinson, Ralph: *Demographic Problems Controversy Over Population Control.* Belmont, Calif., Dickinson Pub. Co. 1967.
2. Among those who qualify for inclusion in this category are Jean Fourastié, Peter Laslett, D.E.C. Eversley, David Glass, T.H. Marshall, Leonard Cain, Norman Ryder, P. Sorokin, J.A. Banks, Maris Vinovskis, Tamara Hareven, and Peter Ulhenberg.
3. Ariès, Philippe: *Western Attitudes Toward Death: From the Middle Ages to the Present.* Baltimore, Md., Johns Hopkins University Press, 1974, pp. 12-15.
4. Ossowski, Stanislaw: *Class Structure in the Social Consciousness.* New York, Free Press, 1963, p. 6.
5. Flinn, M.W.: The stabilization of mortality in pre-industrial western Europe.

The Journal of European History, 3:285, 1974.

6. Ariès, *op. cit.,* pp. 12-13.
7. Solzhenitsyn, Alexander: *The Cancer Ward.* New York, 1969, pp. 96-97.
8. Ariès., *op. cit.,* 1974, p. 13.
9. Uhlenberg, Peter R.: A study of cohort life cycles: cohorts of native born Massachusetts women, 1830-1920. *Population Studies, 23*:414, 1969.
10. Shuddle, Louis O. and Epstein, Lenore A.: Orphanhood — a diminishing problem. *Social Security Bulletin, 18*:17, 1955.
11. Fourastié, Jean: De la vie traditionelle à la vie "tertiare." *Population, 14*:424, 1959.
12. Snow, C.P.: *The Masters,* London, Macmillan, 1951, p. 361.
13. Wolfbein, Seymour: *Employment and Unemployment in the United States: A Study of the American Labor Force,* Chicago, Science Research Asso., 1964, p. 120.
14. Hayflick, Leonard: Perspectives on human longevity. In Neurgarten, Bernice L. and Havighurst, Robert V. (Eds.): *Extending the Human Life Span: Social Policy and Social Ethics.* Chicago, University of Chicago, Committee on Human Development, 1977, p. 1.
15. Dublin, L.I., Lotka, A.J. and Spiegelman, M.: *Length of Life.* New York, Ronald Press, 1949; U.S. Department of Health and Human Services, Public Health Service, *Vital Statistics of the United States,* 1978, Vol. II, Section 5, DHHS Publication No. (PHS) 81-1104, Washington, D.C. 1980.

Chapter 2

A WORLD OF FEAR AND IMMINENT DEATH

UNCONTROLLED disease and premature death haunted people through most of human history. "No thought is born in me that has not 'death' engraved upon it," wrote Michaelangelo.[1] The apparent inevitability of premature death all along the life course resulted in a great familiarity with death. "The spectacle of the dead, whose bones were always being washed up to the surface of the cemeteries, as was the skull of Hamlet, made no more impression upon the living than did the idea of their own death. They were as familiar with the dead as they were familiarized with the idea of their own death."[2]

Much of the art toward the end of the Middle Ages

> reflected a macabre interest in graves and an almost pathological predilection for the manifestations of disease and putrefaction. Countless painters treated with almost loving detail the sufferings of Christ, the terror of the Last Judgment and the tortures of Hell. Woodcuts and paintings depicting the dance of death, inspired directly by the Black Death, enjoyed a morbid popularity. With pitiless realism these paintings portrayed death as a horridly grinning skeleton that seized, without warning, the prince and the peasant, the young and the old, the lovely maiden and the hardened villain, the innocent babe and the decrepit dotard.[3]

Demographically, such dramatic catastrophes as the Black Death were not recurrent enough to keep the average age of death at the level of thirty years. The progress upward, however, was very slow until the latter part of the eighteenth century. In addition to the catastrophic mortality from famine and plague, there was almost constant malnutrition among a large proportion of the population. Diseases such as smallpox, yellow fever, measles, venereal diseases, pneumonia, and tuberculosis contributed to high death rates. Natural disasters such as floods, droughts, torrential rains, crop blights, earthquakes, and the losses incurred from war and rev-

17

olution added to the hazards of life. Human beings appear to have spent much of their lives in fear of death and its related miseries.

"The fundamental characteristic of preindustrial societies was their extreme vulnerability to calamities of all sorts. The most common invocation in preindustrial Europe was '*a bello, fame, et pest libera nos Domine*', (God deliver me from war, famine, and plague). War, famine, and epidemics incessantly caused dramatic peaks of catastrophic mortality."[4]

An excerpt from a letter written by the wife of a doctor living in Iowa appeared at a much later date and gave stark evidence of the pervasive presence of death after the industrial revolution. Monona (Iowa), December 1, 1853, Charlotte to Martha:

> Another year has nearly run its round and perhaps before the close of another some of our number may pass away. I often think of it when I see one after another taken to the graveyard, several families are left to mourn the loss of some of its members. There has been several deaths from small pox in our neighborhood this fall. Some of congestion of the lungs, some of consumption, one man lost and perished on the prairie, so you see there is many ways of hastening us from time to eternity. Our little family still retains a state of tolerable health. . . . (Within four years Charlotte's young son had died, two years later her infant daughter died and four years later she was dead.)[5]

For most men, any hope for the future was almost frivolous in light of the realities of the death rate. Not only was life fortuitous, but disease and starvation frequently led to early disability for those who lived beyond youth. Disability and death were always imminent, and poverty and anonimity were handmaidens. This grisly rhyme has a good deal to say of life and death in the past:

> Rattle his bones, over the stones
> He's only a pauper whom nobody knows.[6]

"When Queen Victoria died at the very outset of the twentieth century, one person in five could expect to come to this, a solitary burial from the workhouse, the poor-law hospital, the lunatic asylum."[7]

Men and women in modern societies are not confronted with their fellow humans' open exhibition of the afflictions and stigma of disease and disaster. Pieter Brueghel's painting, "Carnival Fighting with Lent," no longer has social meaning, other than a curio out of a deep and an unreal past. Most of those depicted in the painting were people with all types of physical and mental deformities — lost limbs, leprosy, scurvy, and apparent mental retardation. Though the afflicted, infirm, and near-dead are still with us, they are shielded more from public view and are not a constant reminder of the tragic side of life.

The decline in premature death over the past two centuries has improved the chances of surviving to a later age for large numbers of people. Data covering the United States from the nineteenth century illustrate the nature of the improvements (*see* Table 2-IV).[8] The greatest gains have occurred in infancy and childhood. In 1840, approximately one fourth of the white males died before their second birthday. By 1890, one fourth of the boys died before the age of seven. In 1910, death took a quarter of the males by approximately age forty-two; and in 1960, 25 percent of the males had died by age seventy-two.

Although the greatest gains in longevity have been made in the early months and years of life, important progress has occurred for the adult ages as well. Between 1840 and 1960, the average remaining lifetime for males at age twenty increased over seventeen years (for females, over twenty years). For cohorts aged forty-five, the average gain in lifetime was over eleven years for men and twelve and one half for women (*see* Table 2-IV). Life has been extended all along the life course.

The decline in premature death was apparent by the middle of the nineteenth century. It was improvements in the general economic and social environment rather than medical science that contributed to improvements in longevity before the twentieth century. Exactly when and how these improvements manifested themselves is impossible to document fully. Adequate scientific data does not usually appear before the middle of the nineteenth century. Nonetheless, there seems to be little doubt that longevity has been improving steadily in many areas throughout the world since around 1750.

Although historical data allows us to assume a general and almost continuous increase in longevity over the past two centuries, the nature and extent of the changes have varied considerably. There were substantial differences in life expectancy between certain small isolated American colonial towns and European countries in the seventeenth century. The early New England villagers were a definite exception in comparison to their European counterparts.[9] These seventeenth century colonial towns enjoyed a standard of life and accompanying health and longevity that compared favorably with present day preindustrial societies. It appears that the better housing, diet, and relative freedom from catastrophic demographic crises account for the exception. These life-saving features resulted in a rapid growth in population compared to the European countries from which they came.[10] Correspondingly, their expected length of life was exceptionally long for this period, when compared to the rest of the world.[11]

Epochs of Catastrophe and Sudden Death

An examination of data on the living conditions from prehistoric to modern times reveals that life was extraordinarily hazardous and brief. The data for accurately ascertaining the length of life prior to the nineteenth century is somewhat inadequate. Nevertheless, the estimates made from written sources, grave inscriptions, and archeological data obtained from examination of mummies and skeletal remains, support the contention that the life expectancies at birth and the average age at death were short by present day standards. Archeological evidence indicates, however, that some men grew old in years, even by modern standards. This has been determined by skeletal remains.

The number and proportion of persons who survive to old age is of crucial concern.[12] Primitive societies in prehistoric times had few, if any, that survived to old age. It has been conjectured that when the old lost their productive capabilities in the past, they were abandoned to die or were killed. It also has been thought that only with the discovery of fire did the old person become of some use, and therefore, allowed to live. Since a fire needed continuous and uninterrupted maintenance "the aged person found protection in it; he still had the strength to help women watch the fire."[13] The increased number of elderly may thus have begun with the rise of civilization itself, a development associated with the discovery and use of fire.

Using preserved skulls acquired from archaeological digs and measuring various features of the skull seams and teeth, data from over 100 Paleolithic remains reveals that not one individual lived to the age of sixty at the time of death.[14] After examining 384 skulls, J.L. Angel estimated that the average age at death ranged between thirty years in neolithic time to thirty-eight years in the Roman period.[15] Karl Pearson, using the labels attached to mummies, calculated life expectancy in Egypt at twenty-two years during Roman times.[16]

Determination of life expectancy in medieval Europe is based on a wide variety of data. In a palaeodemographic study of early (eleventh and twelfth centuries) medieval cemeteries in Hungary, life expectancy at birth was estimated at twenty-nine years. Approximately 50 percent of the population died before reaching twenty-nine. Those who survived to age twenty could only expect to live another twenty-eight years.[17] Whether or not the expected length of life increased during the Middle Ages is almost impossible to answer with any precision. It is estimated that population began increasing in western Europe about the time of the Battle of Hastings, in the middle of the eleventh century. This trend, presumably, continued until about 1350 and can best be accounted for by an improvement in agricultural techniques.[18] A natural increase in population would imply some improvement in overall life expectancy, but not necessarily to late middle or old age. One of the sources of impressionistic information on longevity in this period, was *De Contemptu mundi* (published in 1208), authored by Pope Innocent III. Although hardly qualified as a historical demographer, he stated that "few people reached forty years and those reaching sixty were rare exceptions."[19] Quoting from Eustache Deschamp's work *Miroir de Miriage*, written around 1400, Rosset writes that "people grew old rapidly. Women at the age of thirty were already beginning old age, and for men, old age commenced at fifty."[20] Rosset added that sixty years was the normal end of human life.

Although European populations experienced some growth from ancient times to the high Renaissance, the likelihood of surviving to late middle or early old age was apparently altered very slightly. Population growth was mainly due to improvements in infant mortality. However, the fluctuations in mortality from year to year and country to country were wide and erratic. The record of catastrophic events gives a picture of life in which the level of fear and uncertainty could only have been exceeded by life among primitive men.

Life on the feudal manor may, in retrospect, have seemed peaceful and unharried. Historical evidence, however, reveals a grim existence for most of the inhabitants. Life on the manor was, however, probably better than anywhere else. Poverty, filth, and disease worked in concert to promote an incredibly high level of mortality.

In reconstructing life on a medieval barony, William S. Davis mentions the low level of sanitation, personal cleanliness, and the attendant afflictions and diseases.[21] The peasants were described as people who lived "on the manure heap," and who seldom bathed or washed their rough woolen clothes. The filth brought on skin diseases, the itch, worms, and scrofula, a disease that brought on swelling of lymph glands of the neck. Leprosy was present in many communities. The nature of this dread disease was not understood, and severe (though curable) cases of eczema were sometimes confused with leprosy. Evidence of this misery can be seen in the wooden stave churches of Norway, wherein a special hole in the wall was cut for passing the bread and wine of the Christian communion ceremony to the lepers waiting outside.

As with leprosy, smallpox, cholera, tuberculosis, malaria, rickets, birth defects, and mental disorders were common. "The sufferers from nervous complaints make up small armies. The general terrors and wars of the times, the brooding fears of the devil, hell, and the eternal torment, the spectacle of fearful punishments, and on the other hand, the sheer ennui of life in many castles and in certain ill-ruled convents, drove men and women out of their wits. Such sufferers are lucky if they were treated with kindness and are not, as being 'possessed of devil,' clapped in a dungeon."[22]

For the most part, the healing arts were confined to the barber-surgeon, who provided the semi-annual bleeding of the manor folk. In one case, the local executioner was viewed as an expert surgeon, "since he knows so well how to mutilate bodies, he ought to be able to understand the converse process of curing them."[23] He also had access to a potent remedy, "the fat of a man just hung."

Divine intervention was an important recourse in healing. Prayers to St. Christopher were for indigestion, to St. Roch for the plague, to St. Mathurin for insanity, to St. Rene for kidney complaint, and to St. Crampan for the cramps.[24]

Data on life expectancy in medieval England has been compiled by Russel (*see* Table 2-I). These figures, beginning with estimates of life expectancy before 1276 and encompassing the period of the Black Death in 1348-50, show the grim prospects of an early death all along the life span.[25] Life expectancy at birth varied from seventeen years during the years of the plague, to thirty-five years in the period before 1276. For those who lived to age twenty, life expectancy ranged between a total of forty-two years during 1376-1400 to forty-nine years in 1401-1425. In a study of European ruling families, Peller found that during the years of 1500 to 1699, less than half of the fifteen-year-old boys and girls lived to their fiftieth birthday.[26] These data exemplify the precariousness of life and the normality of early death.

The historical record of life in Europe, from the middle of the fourteenth century until the Industrial Revolution, is filled with evidence of calamity, disaster, and death. Thirteen forty-eight to 1350 saw the pandemic plague, or Black Death.[27] It is believed to have originated in Mesopotamia during the eleventh century, arriving in Constantinople in 1374. It represents one of the monumental events in recorded history. The magnitude of the population loss is hard to fathom, even in the day of thermonuclear bombs and air bombardment. Within three years, Europe had lost one quarter of its population. Though the intensity of the deadly "pest" varied from place to place, few areas escaped the scourge. The population of Florence was reduced from 90,000 to 45,000. Siena lost 15,000 out of 42,000; Hamburg is said to have lost two thirds of its citizens.[28]

Table 2-I

Life Expectancy in Medieval England

AGE	\multicolumn{8}{c}{BIRTH COHORTS}
	Before 1276	1276-1300	1301-1325	1326-1345	1346-1375	1376-1400	1401-1425	1426-1450
0	35.3	31.3	29.8	27.2	17.3	20.5	23.8	32.8
1	40.0	35.8	34.5	31.7	23.7	26.7	28.7	37.0
5	39.9	35.7	34.6	32.3	26.5	28.5	29.4	36.6
10	36.3	32.2	31.0	28.1	25.1	24.5	29.7	34.5
20	28.7	25.2	23.8	22.1	23.9	21.5	29.4	27.7
30	22.8	21.8	20.0	21.1	22.0	22.3	25.0	24.1
40	17.8	16.6	15.7	17.7	18.1	19.2	19.3	20.4
50	12.7	12.3	12.3	14.3	15.9	14.3	14.2	16.4
60	9.4	8.3	9.3	10.8	10.9	10.0	10.5	13.7
70	6.9	6.3	7.0	6.9	6.8	6.3	7.3	10.5
80	5.2	3.8	4.5	6.0	4.7	3.1	4.9	7.9
90	5.0	-	-	2.5	2.5	-	2.5	3.7

Source: Russel, J.C.: Late ancient and medieval population. *Transactions of the American Philosophical Society, 48 (3)*:31, 1958. Reprinted by permission.

From 1348 to 1374, the population of England is estimated to have declined from 3.8 to 2.1 million. In France, the loss of life, augmented by the Hundred Years War, was even greater; Langer states that it took almost two centuries for the population of western and central Europe to regain the size it had been before the Black Death.

For over two centuries, from the fourteenth to well into the sixteenth century, the plague took a heavy toll. The impact of the plague resulted in many extremes of behavior, when people attempted to attribute its cause or escape its ravages. Some attributed it to God's wrath, others to witches, Satan, the physicians, or the Jews. The responses to an outbreak in the community ranged from flagellation to quarantine. All who were financially able fled to the countryside. "At the same time drastic efforts were made to segregate those who were forced to remain in the towns. In the epidemic of 1563, Queen Elizabeth took refuge in Windsor Castle and had a gallows erected on which to hang anyone who had the temerity to come out to Windsor from plague-ridden London."[29] Troops were used to cordon off an infected town, letting no one in or out. Quarantines were enforced by chaining off whole streets and building gallows as a warning to those who might violate the regulations. "The French surgeon, Ambroise Paré, writing of the plague epidemic in 1568, reported that husbands and wives deserted each other, that parents sometimes even abandoned their children and that people went mad with terror and committed suicide."[30]

After the Black Death of 1345-50, rural economies collapsed in many places. Death in rural areas was so great that few were left to till the land, and most or all of the artisans died or moved away. A surviving youth might become sole owner of a large manor, with no knowledge of farming and few tenants. Whole areas were abandoned as a result of the plague. A significant proportion of the population moved to the towns and cities; many of the institutional features of medieval Europe, such as agriculture and serfdom, were drastically altered. The demand for labor was so great that serfdom suffered a sharp decline. "The surviving labourers sought work where they could command the best wages and at the same time could escape from the few degrading bonds of servitude which still clung to . . . the serfs of a manor."[31] The collapse of life in many rural areas eventually gave impetus to urban growth, but a full scale urbanization of western Europe would not take place for over 200 years. In 1800, most of the world's population still consisted of peasants, approximately 80 to 90 percent of the population in Europe.[32]

Though the bubonic plague never again reached the pandemic proportions of 1384, many serious epidemics occurred during the next few centuries. Urban areas seemed particularly vulnerable, though small towns were not immune. Venice declined from 170,000 in 1556 to 120,000 in 1577 due to the plague. Genoa lost 30,000 of its 70,000 population between 1656 and 1660.[33] At an even later date, local archives reveal data on the death toll of a smallpox epidemic. Death claimed 300 per thousand in Copenhagen in 1711, 450 per thousand in Danzig in 1709, and 500 per thousand in Toulon in 1720.[34] As late as 1771, Moscow lost over 56,000 lives to bubonic plague, almost a fourth of the population.[35]

The plague struck Marseilles in the summer of 1720.[36] The violence of the epidemic is illustrated by the fact that of the 80,000 people remaining in the city, almost 40,000 died. Ten thousand had fled before the city was cordoned off from the countryside. Food preparation, as well as other services, was seriously impaired. In late summer, almost all of the millers, bakers, and butchers had died or fled. "All policemen, all captains except one, all lieutenants except two, all public servants (almost five hundred), . . . and almost all of the three hundred and fifty men of the company of guards died. In the health services, of the twelve doctors who remained, six contracted the plague and four died; of the thirty-five surgeons, thirty-two died."[37] Among various artisans, the death toll exceeded 50 percent. Of an estimated 134 carpenters, eighty-four died; of 138 tailors, seventy-eight died; of 200 shoemakers, 111 died; of 400 cobblers, 350 died; and of 500 masons, thirty-five died. An account states that "volunteers gathered together twelve to thirteen hundred infants who had lost their mothers and tried to nourish them with soup and goat's milk. The babies died at the rate of thirty or forty a day."[38]

Over a century later, Asiatic or Indian cholera had made its way from Bengal across Asia to England. The British had been free of major epidemic diseases for a long period when this disease struck. Cholera was to have an effect far beyond that of diseases like small pox or tuberculosis. "It was . . . a disease capable of inducing sheer blind panic, for it struck swiftly and savagely, leaving havoc, pain and distress in its wake."[39]

Though the statistics of diseases and their consequences are scanty and subject to considerable error, early attempts were made to develop life tables for estimating the average years of survival of various age-groups. The results provide a further glimpse of the deathly nature of preindustrial society. John Graunt's early life table, computed for London about 1660, reveals that of every 100 infants, only six survived to their fifty-sixth year and three to their sixth-sixth.[40] In contrast, the astronomer Halley, found in his life table for Wroclaw, that 19 percent of each cohort born survived to their sixty-fifth year.[41]

Through the use of a similar type of retrospective data and calculation, Mallet found that in Geneva, out of every 100 infants, the following numbers survived to the 60th year:[42]

16th century	8.6
17th century	14.9
18th century	25.9[43]

The Normality of Hunger and Starvation: Past and Present

The historical record is filled with heroes and heroines and their memorable moments, but little is recorded regarding the time and energy our ancestors spent in their quest for food. Although pestilence was a major element in causing misery, uncertainty, and a short life, the lack of nourishing food and poor sanitary conditions may have been more important in determining the reasons for the slow rise in longevity. Like the diseases that become pandemic, hunger frequently attained similar proportions, often reaching the level of famine. The relationship between famine and epidemics is often reciprocal. Famine, a slow but effective killer, has been much more common in the past than most of us realize.

In their impressive study of human starvation, Professor Ancel Keys and his associates attempted to list some of the "notable famines in history."[44] They noted that famines have usually been defined in terms of drastic fluctuations in food prices plus the activity of governmental authorities in requisitioning food and distributing it to the public. It appears as though hunger was so commonplace and such an integral part of life that it was not necessary to mention it in the literature of the past. "Horrible episodes that brought the death of one out of five living beings are passed by in silence while every detail is given about the marriage of the Dauphin, the disgrace of a minister or a mistress."[45]

Keys' listing of famines, with the exception of India, is very incomplete except for the British Isles, Northwestern Europe, and the Mediterranean Basin. The tabulation omits local famines, long periods of food shortage that did not reach famine conditions, and famines that were directly caused by looting and pillaging in wartime. Despite such omissions, the list is chilling; of the 229 famines listed from the eighth to the twentieth centuries, only twenty-two of them were outside of Europe. Other sources provide additional data: "Cornelius Walford listed over 200 famines between the year A.D. 1 and 1850 in the territories now comprising Great Britain alone. Over the same period, there were 2,000 famines in China, almost one a year. It has been estimated that between five and ten million have died during famines in the twentieth century."[46] Although the definition of famine and the reliability of the early data is problematic, it is clear that shortage of food was a major element in the life of the past.

Table 2-II

The Number of Notable Famines Outside of India

Century	Number of Famines
8th	12
9th	19
10th	15
11th	24
12th	23
14th	20
15th	13
16th	18
17th	10
18th	21
19th	25
20th	6

Source: Keys, Ancel B. et al.: *The Biology of Human Starvation*, Vol. II, Minneapolis, University of Minnesota Press, 1950, pp. 1247-1252.

As is abundantly evident, the crisis of subsistence has swept the world through most of human history. Although the Malthusian theory was generally confirmed by evidence throughout Europe, countries like England seemed to experience death by starvation a little less than some of the other countries. Nevertheless, direct evidence of it appears from the mortality records of Greystoke in the cumberland hills of England:

"Extracts from the Register of Greystoke 1623

29th January:	'A poor fellow destitute of succour and was brought out of the street in Johnby into the house of Anthony Clemmerson, constable there, where he died.'
27th March:	'A poor hungerstarved beggar child, Dorothy, daughter of Henry Patteson, Miller.'
28th March:	'Thomas Simpson, a poor hungerstarved beggar boy and son of one Richard Simpson of Brough by Mandgyes house in Throp.'
19th May:	At night, 'James Irwin, a poor beggar stripling born upon the bourders of England. He died in Johnby in great misery.'
12th July:	'Thomas, child of Richard Bell, a poor man, which child died for very want of food and maintenance to live.'
11th September:	'Leonard, son of Anthony Cowlman, of Johnby late deceased, which child died for want of food and maintence to live.'
12th September:	'Janie, wife of Anthony Cowlman, late deceased which woman died in Edward Dawson's barn of Greystoke for want of maintence.'
27th September:	'John, son of John Lancaster, late of Greystoke, a waller by trade, which child died for want of food and means.' (The register tells us that he was baptized on October 17th, 1619, so he was four years old.)
4th October:	Agnes, wife of John Lancaster, late of Greystoke, a waller by his trade, which woman died for want of means to life.'
27th October:	'William, child of Lancelot Brown, which Lancelot went forth of the country (the district) for want of means.' "[47]

In the nineteenth century, an epic famine took place in Ireland.[48] The human misery and devastation suffered by millions of Irishmen between 1845 and 1849 is incomprehensible. Massive death from starvation resulted from the potato blight, which has not been experienced since in western Europe. Rough estimates indicate that about two and one half million people were lost due to famine and the accompanying assaults of disease.[49] No accurate records of deaths were kept. Death not only took place on the roads and byways, but entire families died and remained in their mud huts for days before being discovered. The victims were buried in ditches or mass graves, few memories and no records remaining. In the four provinces of Ireland, the smallest population loss was 15.5 percent in Leinster; the largest loss was Connaought, with a 28.6 percent loss.[50]

Hunger, and its ravages, were not new to Ireland at the time of the great potato famine. The British Poor Inquiry Commission reported that over two million persons, in a population of about eight million, suffered from starvation every year. In attempting to relieve the situation imposed by the destruction of one potato crop after another, the British government had to contend with endemic hunger. "This hopeless, wretched, multitude, already starving, already diseased, unemployed beggars, dispossessed squatters, evicted persons, penniless widows, starving children, snatched at every offer of relief, swamped every scheme, and formed a hard core of destitution whose numbers could be reduced only by death."[51]

Although Ireland was not among the leaders in the industrial revolution, life had eased for some and the average life expectancy had increased. Although industrialization was underway at the time of the famine, poverty and destitution continued to be the hand-maiden of death to a degree that had been largely prevented among modern industrial nations.[52] " 'The outstanding feature of mortality behaviour in Western Europe in all centuries before the twentieth has been a great instability.' "[53]

Using historical records and analyzing the findings in terms of the concept of *level of living,* Fourastié has provided data on the extreme fluctuations in the economic situation of the masses in France and in other parts of Europe in the eighteenth century. "After 1709, the demographic expansion of the western nations was progressively freed from the millennial rhythm of the famines. The brutal saw teeth of the old mortality excesses of famine years, formerly the predominant factor in demography and the sole determinant of population disappear. . . ."[54]

During the eighteeth century, France grew from eighteen or twenty million to twenty-seven million.[55] The level of living differed from what it had been in previous times. The fluctuations, based largely on the relationship of the price of food grains to the level of wages, were less pronounced than they had been in the past. Though malnutrition and hunger probably did occur, it was diminished in severity and magnitude. Fourastié quotes the Englishman, Arthur Young, who described conditions before the French Revolution in the *Voyage in France*.

Young was impressed with the poverty-ridden level of existence. In describing workers' homes in Savoy he wrote, "The houses have a repulsive aspect . . . they are huts of mud, ugly, covered with straw, smoke escaping from a hole in the roof or even from the windows. Window glass seems to be unknown and these houses have an air of poverty which clashes with the general appearance of the countryside."[56] This was the period in which the "King of France could feed his workmen with two daily pounds of millet bread, a quart of wine and two bowls of gravy soup, *sometimes fat, sometimes lean.*"[57]

For most of man's existence in the temperate zones of the world, the seasons mirrored the level of subsistence. The autumn of the year was a time of plenty, but by the end of winter, all but the rich began to experience hunger. The availability of surplus food in some parts of the world, in addition to the technology of storage and preservation, is a recent development. The process for the canning of food was invented in France in 1809. It reached the United States in 1820.[58] Freezing as a method of preservation was initiated in the early years of the twentieth century and has been fully developed only since World War II. Large-scale efficient storage of grain and food stuffs has been linked with the production of surpluses; this is basically a phenomenon of modern times. Despite the new technology, the problem of getting enough to eat remains a paramount concern for many.

Though the threat of famine has been diminished in the industrial countries, it continues to occur in the underdeveloped nations. Hunger remains a common experience in the lives of most men on earth. In an investigation on the state of nutrition throughout the world in 1952, the Food and Agricultural Organization of the United Nations found that only 28 percent of the world's population had access to a calorically sufficient diet.[59]

Of greater importance is the "hidden hunger" of protein deficiency. The Food and Agricultural Organization found that only 17 percent of the world's population consumed a diet adequate in protein (1.058 ounces of animal protein per day); 58 percent live on less than half this required amount. Along with these deficiencies in calories and protein, other essential nutritional deficiencies in vitamins, amino acids, minerals, and fats also occur. With the growth of biological science and nutrition, many unseen and disguised consequences of nutritional inadequacies are coming to light. The precise nutritional needs for the maintenance of essential body functions and a high level of vigor and well-being are still hotly contested. There is, however, little doubt that dietary deficiencies are common everywhere, though they are a significant factor in premature death only in the undeveloped countries.

Pellagra, beriberi, scurvy, pernicious anemia, and xerophthalmia were common diseases of nutritional inadequacy. Little was known about these diseases until the nineteenth century; they have taken a countless toll of lives throughout antiquity and the middle ages. Biological deterioration associated with hunger is "actually capable of reducing the organism to a state of relative incapacity, of feeble productivity, and of attenuated resistance to a whole body of other diseases that pounce on the enfeebled organism."[60] Diseases such as tuberculosis, trachoma, leprosy, and gastro-intestinal parasitoses count heavily against the underfed. De Castro argues that although not the determining factor in disease, "defective nutrition is the predominant factor" in disease.[61]

Though the science of nutrition is embryonic in comparison to the more pathogenic approach of medicine, hunger and undernourishment play a role in disease and premature death. Various forms of debility and physical incapacity are related to poor nutrition, especially in old people. With adequate diet and modern medicine, the speed at which the older age cohorts are depleted tends to decline. The rate of depletion of each cohort has social and social psychological consequences of which we are not yet fully aware. Greater longevity and the full development of gerontology will help create an awareness of the consequences of health and aging. Long life requires greater emphasis on the nutritional needs in maintaining the highest level of physical and mental functioning through middle and old age.[62]

Longevity and Medical Science

By 1850, it was apparent to many people in Europe and the United States that death rates were declining. A basic cause for this decrease is not determinable, although the uninformed have frequently attributed it to the marvels of modern medical science. Medical science did not really emerge until after 1850. Before that, medicine was, at best, a craft. When William Jenner took his diploma in medicine in 1837, the tools of the trade were a scalpel for blood-letting and a wooden stethoscope. He had neither a clinical thermometer and few if any effective drugs.

In attempting to isolate the causes of the declining death rate, some modern scholars conclude that medical treatments have had little, if any effect. McKeown and Brown state that "The decline in the death rate during the nineteenth century was almost wholly attributable to environmental change, and owed little to specific therapy, preventive or curative (an exception to this was vaccination against smallpox)."[63]

Dubos states the following:

> Because the decrease in death rates appeared obvious to everyone after 1900, scientific medicine, and the germ theory in particular have been given all the credit for the general health of the people. The present generation goes still further and now believes that the control of infectious disease dates from the widespread use of antibacterial drugs. . . .In truth, the mortality of many other infections had begun to recede in Western Europe and North America long before the introduction of specific methods of therapy, indeed before the demonstration of the germ theory of disease.[64]

Changes occurring in eighteenth century London illustrate the nature of some of the contributions to the postponement of death. Many of these changes may be attributable to the new thoughtways and perspectives associated with the Enlightenment. An awareness of the tremendous waste of human life through disease and death led to the establishment of lying-in hospitals and dispensaries for the poor. New attitudes toward the hygienic value of fresh air and cleanliness and the deleterious effects of gin drinking emerged in this period. The paving of streets, digging of sewers, development of winter fodder for cattle, and better ways of food preservation ushered in a new era of living conditions.

The foundling hospitals, as well as lying-in hospitals, were created in order to curb the number of cases of infants dying from exposure, desertion, and outright murder. The high rates of infant death among the poor brought about the latter. New knowledge of childbearing developed. The dispensary movement brought doctors into intimate contact with the health problems of the poor.

"Creighton has pointed out that medical practice in the eighteenth century lay chiefly among the richer classes, and that the physicians knew little of the state of health in the cellars and tenement houses. The dispensary doctors knew a great deal, and had a double effect, resulting in a cumulative improvement in the health of London: the poor learned something of the rudiments of hygiene, the doctors learned how to diagnose the diseases of poverty and dirt; the richer classes began to hear of the conditions under which the poor lived."[65]

During the eighteenth century, gin drinking reached disastrous proportions. In the 1720s it was reported that every tenth house in London was engaged in selling some kind of liquor.[66] Gin drinking was joined with poverty and accentuated the tremendous waste of life, both in the death of the young and in the misery of those who believed that liquor was beneficial. By midcentury, much had been done to diminsh the indiscriminate use of alcohol.

Sanitation, new ways of food preparation, and the use of cotton for clothing contributed to improved health. Paving the street and using the refuse as manure for agriculture improved sanitation. The development of winter fodder for cattle was important; fodder allowed the farmer to keep his cattle alive during the winter, thereby reducing the necessity of living on salted meats during half of the year. As mentioned earlier, canning was discovered in the early nineteenth century. This method of food preservation laid the basis for new and improved diets throughout the industialized world. Finally, the manufacture of cheap cotton cloth became a reality after midcentury. Before then, much of the clothes were seldom if ever washed, especially among the poor. A journeyman's or tradesman's wife might wear leather stays and a quilted petticoat until they virtually rotted away. The new cheap cotton garments could easily be washed, which increased cleanliness and fostered better health.

Though these changes were occurring in places like London, they were largely tangential to the practice of medicine. Most of the contributions to longevity were related to the change in the social and economic environment of the destitute and poor. By midcentury, the level of living had been stabilized and began to rise despite the negative features of early industrialization.

Rising from forty years in 1850, to sixty plus in 1940, the recent increase in life expectancy in the industrialized West was the result of nonmedical developments, although immunization did have important effects. Akerknect, a historian of medicine, wrote the following: "miraculous and admirable as the new antibiotics . . . may be, they have never saved nearly as many lives as the rather prosaic procedure of pasteurizing milk. Oliver Wendell Holmes once said: 'The bills of mortality are more affected by drainage than this or that method of medical practice.' "[67] Though debatable, statements like these have gained the stature of truisms in the writings of historical demographers.

During the Romantic period in the nineteenth century, death among youth gained increased attention in the literary world. At this time, tuberculosis was an important cause of debilitation and death. The emphasis on youth and the prevalence of the White Plague combined to make men and women very much aware of the precariousness and brevity of life. "This was the time when, in Keats words, 'Youth grows pale, spectre thin and dies.' The fading away of young women dying of consumption — in a decline, as it is proper to say — became a poetical theme of literature.' . . . The tragic atmosphere pervading the novels of the Brontë sisters reflects the prevalence of disease all around them. The four sisters and their brothers died consumptive in their youth or early adulthood."[68]

The ravages of a deadly disease have had decided effects on the rise of science. In the 1930s, cholera reached pandemic proportions in Europe and most of the rest of the world. Akerknect wrote, "Cholera was once called our best ally in the fight for better hygiene. Its dramatic effects frightened legislators into taking progressive measures far more rapidly than the creeping death resulting from tuberculosis or typhoid."[69]

Although the late nineteenth century marked the beginning of a new era in the control over death, the state of public hygiene remained inadequate for years to come. In the United States, diarrheal diseases took a heavy toll on infants during hot summer months.[70] An important cause was the lack of sanitation in the handling of milk. A study conducted in New York City noted that many dairies kept their milk in dirty containers.[71] Milk was transported into the city in five and ten gallon cans. Bottled milk did not become available until the 1920s. Mechanical refrigeration was not well developed until the 1930s and 40s. Prior to that, the family's milk pail was kept outside the window on the fire escape or in an inefficient ice box.

The prebacteriological sanitation movement was essentially a fight against filth and stench. Although the causal agents of many of the diseases were unknown, the movement inadvertently did a great deal toward removing or inhibiting many of the causal factors. It concentrated on a fight against water pollution, insufficient sewers, overcrowded housing, adulterated foods, and child labor. In 1848, the British enacted the Public Health Act, the Nuisances Removal and Diseases Prevention Acts, and established the General Board of Health. At the time of the health acts, Britain lost 54,000 people from an out break of cholera. Through the work of the Board of Health, it was deduced that cholera was spread by polluted drinking water and prompt measures were taken.

During the middle of the nineteenth century, scientific developments occurred in rapid succession. The slow but steady acceptance of the germ theory of disease was a major step in the control of death. Although bacteria had been studied as early as the eighteenth century, it was the genius of Louis Pasteur (1822-1895) and subsequently Robert Koch (1843-1910) that established the modern science of bacteriology. In 1885, Pasteur produced a vaccine that was effective against rabies. Koch, in a similar fashion, advanced the development of bacteriology.

These scientific developments marked the real beginning of effective disease control by medical science:

It is impossible to overemphasize the importance of the fact that for the first time in history *causes* of numerous diseases became known, the way was opened for a replacement of symptomatic or empirical treatment with causal treatment and prevention. A definite answer could finally be given to the question as to whether the disease-producing agent was a 'miasma,' a chemical agent, or a living organism. The problem of the specificity of diseases was solved. The gap between the discoveries of pure science and their successful application in practice was bridged faster than ever before. This fact impressed the lay public with the potentialities of medicine more than any previous discovery. Rational treatment and prevention of infectious diseases became possible on an unprecedented scale. The whole of medicine was transformed, with the fields of public health and surgery undergoing complete rejuvenation.[72]

At this juncture in the history of medicine, the work of Lister and others advanced the principle of asepsis (the use of sterile instruments and dressings) in surgery. By preventing wound infection after surgery, the stage was set for the development of an adequate anesthetic. In 1846, a famous operation took place at Massachusetts

General Hospital in which ether was used successfully as a pain killer. By controlling infection and pain, surgery moved steadily toward such twentieth century spectaculars as open heart, brain surgery, and organ transplants.

The developments in bacteriology, chemistry, physiology, and medical technology occurred at an accelerated rate at the beginning of the twentieth century. Though destroying a large proportion of a generation of European men, the First World War also gave medical science a forward boost. A new attack on disease and preventive death began a few years before the Second World War broke out. Antibiotics first appeared in 1935 with the discovery of sulfa drugs. These were followed in quick succession by penicillin (1941), streptomycin (1944), Chloromycetin® (1948), and Aureomycin® (1949). This potent array of drugs has conquered many of the infectious diseases including tuberculosis, typhoid fever, cholera, pneumonia, and venereal diseases.

The years of World War II brought the full development of the highly effective pesticide, DDT. Thus far, DDT may have saved more lives than all the antibiotics combined, through the eradication of disease carrying insects such as the anopheles mosquito. Paradoxically, this highly effective pesticide now appears to pose a serious threat to human health and the natural environment.

The health and welfare of thousands of people has also been improved by the synthesis and manufacture of a number of glandular secretions. Insulin, adrenalin, folliculin, and cortisone serve to replace or supplement the products of glands such as the pancreas, ovaries, and the thymus. The advancement of knowledge about the subtle interrelationships within the endocrine system has progressed, but it has a great distance to go before its full role in the prolongation of life is determined.

Physicists and engineers have contributed to radiation therapy, electro-magnetic waves, mechanical hearts and kidneys, electronic pacemakers, new prosthetic devices and a multiplicity of tools and instruments for diagnosis and therapy. Though not all of the developments have added directly to the prolongation of life, they have often reduced suffering of the afflicted.

As a result of the advancements in the health sciences, a considerable number of people who under earlier conditions would have died in childhood, youth, and middle age are still living. These were lives that would not have been saved by the improvements in sewers, water purification, sanitation in food production, or adequate diet. Modern bacteriology and the so-called miracle drugs gave the latest push to increased longevity, and eliminated a great deal of uncertainty surrounding illness and disease.

The improvement in life expectancy resulted primarily from a reduction in infant mortality due to pasteurization, pure water, and hygiene. Following the victories over infant death, any new improvements would necessarily have a much smaller effect on the average length of life. It is a dramatic observation that the expected length of life jumped from thirty years in the period before modern science to seventy years at the present time. The fact that this gain was mostly a result of the decline in infant mortality has frequently obscured its social importance.

It is one of the functions of this investigation to call attention to recent increases in longevity (since 1750) by emphasizing that currently living cohorts have been given substantial increments of additional living time in contrast to those who went through the life course in the past. The French demographer, Sauvy, has developed data on the comparative survival rates for various age levels during different historical times for several widely varying populations. These data reveal the numbers who survived through the life span in France before mortality rates declined in India, an underdeveloped country, and in Norway, a fully developed country, in the midtwentieth century. Comparing modern Norway with eighteeth century France (Norway probably shared France's survival rate in the eighteenth century), the number in Norway surviving to age twenty would have almost doubled (502 to 950). Those surviving to age forty was even greater in numbers (369 to 916). The prospect of a future increase in longevity for India is illustrated by a comparison with Norway at midcentury. In 1950, Norway had a survival rate to age forty that was twice as high as that of India.

A great qualitative change has taken place in the social and psychological milieu of birth cohorts passing through the life course in modern societies. According to an American demographer, "The countries with the greatest average duration of life have by now about exhausted the possibility of increasing survivorship in a way that makes for a younger population. In Sweden, 95 percent survive from birth to age thirty, compared to 67 percent in 1870."[73] In 1978,

Table 2-III

Comparative Survival Rates

	France (18th century)	India (1941-1950)	Norway (1946-1950)
		Number of Survivors	
At birth	1000	1000	1000
1 year	767	818	970
20 years	502	574	950
40 years	369	422	916
60 years	214	216	818
80 years	35	27	388
85 years	12	2	214

Source: Sauvy, Alfred: *Fertility and Survival,* New York, Criterion Books, 1961, p. 40.

in the United States, "75 percent of the infants born . . . will reach sixty-five; of those who do, they will live, on the average, for another sixteen years, to age eighty-one."[74] The timing of death has made a radical shift in the recent history of the world. Life expectancy is getting so close to the human lifespan that further improvements will be slow and difficult. Lifespan is generally believed to be approximately a hundred years. For example, if cancer as a cause of death was completely eliminated, the increase in life expectancy at birth, in modern societies, would be only two to three years.[75] Sauvy comments on this development: "Until only very recently, longevity remained more or less the same. Leaving aside periods of war, we can find no essential differences between prehistoric men, the men of ancient times and those of predevelopment modern times. A stone that has weighed upon the human race for aeons has now been lifted."[76]

A more recent body of data (Table 2-IV) provides a comparison on longevity for each decade from 1840-1960. These data reveal the important gains made for the American adult population. The average remaining lifetime for a cohort of males at age twenty in 1840 was forty-one years; and in 1960 for the twenty-year-old cohort it was fifty-eight, an increase of seventeen years. For the cohorts at age forty-five, the gain during the same period was eleven years. For women, the gains were greater by two or three years. "Between the 1840 and 1960 cohorts, the average remaining lifetime at age forty-five will have increased about eleven years among white men and twelve and one half years among white women; at age sixty-five, the corresponding gains will be over six years and seven years. As a con-

Table 2-IV

The Average Remaining Lifetime (in Years) at Specific Ages for
White Males and Females in the United States
By Year of Birth From 1840 to 1960

Year of Birth	Age in Years					Year of Birth	Age in Years				
	0	5	20	45	65		0	5	20	45	65
Male						**Female**					
1840	38.7	51.8	41.3	24.1	11.6	1840	40.8	51.6	41.4	25.4	12.3
1850	41.6	52.4	41.6	24.5	11.8	1850	43.8	52.9	42.1	26.0	12.6
1860	44.3	53.0	42.0	24.8	11.8	1860	45.9	53.9	43.6	26.7	12.9
1870	44.0	54.0	43.3	25.7	12.4	1870	46.8	56.2	46.1	28.1	14.1
1880	46.3	55.9	44.7	26.2	12.9	1880	50.1	59.5	48.6	29.8	15.4
1890	48.0	58.2	46.0	26.8	13.2	1890	53.2	63.3	51.2	31.6	16.3
1900	53.4	60.6	48.6	27.9	14.0	1900	59.8	66.4	54.2	33.4	17.3
1910	57.8	63.6	50.8	29.3	14.8	1910	64.8	69.8	56.9	34.8	17.9
1920	63.1	65.6	52.3	30.8	15.5	1920	70.8	72.6	59.1	35.8	18.2
1930	67.7	68.5	54.7	32.0	15.8	1930	74.2	74.3	60.2	36.5	18.4
1940	70.1	70.2	56.1	32.9	16.2	1940	76.7	75.3	60.9	36.8	18.7
1950	73.9	71.6	57.3	33.9	16.9	1950	78.9	76.2	61.5	37.3	19.1
1960	75.7	73.0	58.6	35.2	17.8	1960	80.1	77.0	62.3	38.0	19.5

Reprinted from: Jacobson, Paul H.: Cohort survival for generations since 1840. *The Millbank Memorial Fund Quarterly, 42 (3)*:48, 1968, by permission of the MIT Press, Cambridge, Massachusetts. Copyright© 1968 by the MIT Press.

Note: The above table is a generation life table, whereas the life tables readily available from the Bureau of Census are current life tables. On the current life table for 1978, the life expectancy at age 65, for example, varies from the above figures from 1.1 to 3.8 years for whites.

sequence, when the 1960 cohort attains age sixty-five in 2025, the men will be able to look forward to seventeen and three-fourths additional years of life, on the average, while women will still have an average of nineteen and one-half years ahead of them,"[77] Jacobson's estimates can only be fully confirmed when the various cohorts involved have died, it appears that the projections in Table 2-IV will be "fairly close to experience."[78]

Although the prolongation of life is of great importance, it is the accompanying awareness of the decrease in the imminence of death and the uncertainty surrounding disease and morbidity that are the keys to great change in human life.

Though the data detailing the changes in the pattern of death and the increases in longevity are sketchy and limited for the eighteenth and nineteenth centuries, it is clear a major change in the circumstances of the life and death of modern men and women has taken place. The human community's earlier concerns with pandemic disease, famine, disaster, and high rates of premature death gave life a temporary quality infused with fear and uncertainty. Improvements in the general conditions of life, particularly in higher incomes, diet, personal hygiene, public health, sanitation, and the development of scientific medicine, have wrought profound changes in the chronology of death. How this new chronology has affected the life perspective and social consciousness of men and women in modern society will be discussed in the next chapter.

REFERENCES

1. Quoted by Langer, William L.: The black death. *Scientific American, 210*:121, 1964.
2. Ariès, Philippe: *Western Attitudes Toward Death: From the Middle Ages to the Present,* translated by Patricia M. Ranum. Baltimore, The John Hopkins University Press, 1974, p. 25.
3. Cippola, Carlo M.: *Before the Industrial Revolution: European Society and Economy, 1000-1700.* New York, W.W. Norton, 1976, p. 151.
4. William L. Langer, *op. cit,* p. 121.
5. Coffin, Margaret M.: *Death in Early America.* Nashville Tenn., Thomas Nelson, Inc., 1976, pp. 55 ff.
6. Laslett, Peter: *The World We Have Lost.* London, Methuen, 1965, p. 200.
7. *Ibid.*
8. The following data and comparisons were developed by Jacobson, Paul H.: Cohort survival for generations since 1840. *The Milbank Memorial Fund Quarterly, 42, 3*:43ff, 1964. The data used in subsequent paragraphs was quoted from this study.
9. Lockridge, Kenneth A.: *A New England Town: The First Hundred Years.* Dedham, Mass., 1636-1736. New York, W.W. Norton, 1970; Demos, John: *A Little Commonwealth: Family Life in Plymouth Colony.* New York, Oxford University Press, 1970; Greuen, Philip, Jr.: *Four Generations: Population, Land and family in Colonial Andover,* Massachusetts. Ithaca, New York, 1970; Norton, Susan L.: Population growth in colonial America: a study of Ipswich, Massachusetts. *Population Studies, 25*:433-452, 1971; Smith, Daniel S.: The demographic history of New England. *Journal of Economic History, 32*:165-183, 1972; Vinovskis, Maris A.: American historical demography: a review essay. *Historical Methods Newsletter, 4*:141-148, 1971; and Vinovskis, Maris A.: Mortality rates and trends in Massachusetts before 1860. *Journal of Economic History, 32*:184-213, 1972.
10. Lockridge, Kenneth A.: The population of Dedham, Massachusetts, 1636-1736. *The Economic History Review, 19 (2)*:329, 1966.
11. According to Demos, life expectancies in late 17th century Plymouth Colony

were

Age	Men	Women
21	69.2	62.4
30	70.0	64.7
40	71.2	69.7
50	73.7	73.4
60	76.3	76.8
70	79.9	80.7
80	85.1	86.7

These data are based on a sample of 654 persons.
Source: Demos, John: *A Little Commonwealth: Family Life in Plymouth Colony*. New York, Oxford University Press, 1970, p. 192.

12. Official and scholarly definitions of "old age" have generally put its onset at 60 or 65 years.
13. Krzywicki, L.: *Ludy Zarys Anthropologic Etniczny*. (Nations Outline of Ethic Anthropology). Warshaw, 1893, p. 47, quoted by Rosset, Edward: *Aging Process of Population*, New York, MacMillan, 1964, p. 104.
14. *Ibid.*, p. 105.
15. Angel, J. Lawrence: The length of life in ancient Greece. *Journal of Gerontology*, 2:1824, 1947.
16. Pearson, Karl: On the change in expectation of life in man during the period of circa 2000 years. *Biometrika*, (1901-02), pp. 261-264; McConnell, W.R.: On the expectation of life in ancient Rome and in the provinces of Hispania and Lusitania and Africa. *Biometrika* 9:366-380, 1913. The variations in these figures connote the general inadequacy of the data.
17. Acsádi, G. and Nemeskéri, J.: *History of Human Life Span and Mortality*. Budapest, Akadémiai Kiadó, 1970, pp. 250-51.
18. Genicot, Leopold: *Countours of Middle Ages*, translated by Lawrence and Lora Wood. London, Routledge and Kegan Paul, 1967, p. 132-33.
19. Quoted by Russet, *op. cit.*, p. 110.
20. *Ibid.*, p. 110; Rosset cautions us that Deschamps was an avid hater of women, hence his declaration of such an early age for the aging of women may be suspect. However, he feels that his estimate for men may be quite valid, especially since he was 70 years old when he wrote *Mirror of Marriage*.
21. Davis, William Sterns: *Life in a Medieval Barony: A Picture of a Typical Feudal Community in the Thirteenth Century*. New York, Harpers, 1923, p. 278.
22. *Ibid.*, p. 279.
23. *Ibid.*, p. 280.
24. *Ibid.*, p. 279-280.
25. Russel, J.C.: Late ancient and medieval population, *Transactions of the American Philosphical Society*, 48:31, 1958.
26. Peller, Sigismund: Mortality, past, and future. *Population Studies*, 1(4)·429, 1948.
27. Langer, William: The black death. *Scientific American*, 210:114-115, 1964.
28. Unless otherwise referred, the figures in this section are from Langer, *Ibid.*

29. *Ibid.*, p. 116.
30. *Ibid.*, pp. 116-117.
31. Creighton, Charles: *History of Epidemics in England*, Vol. I. New York, Barnes and Noble, 1965, p. 182 ff.
32. Fourastié, Jean: Predicting economic changes in our times. *Diogenes, 5*:1954.
33. Reinhard, Marcel and Armengaud, Andre: *Histoire Générale de la Population Mondiale.* Paris, Editions Montchrestien, 1961, p. 86, 145.
34. Fourastié, *op. cit.,* p. 230.
35. Alexander, John T.: Catherine II, bubonic plague and the problems of industry in Moscow. *The American Historical Review, 79:*1974.
36. The following account is taken from Biraben, Jean-Noel: Certain demographic characteristics of the plague epidemic in France, 1720-1722, from Glass, D.V. and Revelle, Roger (Eds.): *Population and Social Change*, London, Edward Arnold, 1972, pp. 234-236.
37. *Ibid.*, p. 235.
38. *Ibid.*, p. 234.
39. Duney, Michael: *The Return of the Plague: British Society and the Cholera 1831-1832.* Dublin, Gil and Macmillan, 1979, p. 2.
40. Westergaard, Harold L.: *Contributions to the History of Statistics.* London, P.A. King and Son, 1932, p. 22.
41. Rosset, *op. cit.,* p. 115.
42. *Ibid.*, p. 117.
43. This is not meant to ignore the general fact that infant deaths have been high throughout most of human history, irrespective of the vagaries of diet or food supplies. Hunger and famine has affected longevity all along the life course of our forebearers as well as many of our contemporaries.
44. Keys, Ancel B., et al.: *The Biology of Human Starvation*, Vol., II. Minneapolis, University of Minnesota Press, 1950, pp. 1247-1252.
45. Fourastié, Jean: *The Causes of Wealth,* translated and edited by Theodore Caplow. Glencoe, Ill., The Free Press, 1960, p. 61-62.
46. Parsons, Jack: *Population Fallicies.* London, Elek/Pemberton, 1977, p. 31.
47. Laslett, *op. cit.,* p. 115.
48. Woodham Smith, Cecil, did in fact, produce an epic in *The Great Hunger,* New York, New American Library, 1962.
49. *Ibid.*, p. 409.
50. *Ibid.*, p. 409.
51. *Ibid.*, p. 160.
52. Important famines did occur however, in China in 1877, 1916, and 1929, with losses running into the millions. Russia has also experienced no less than ten famines since the great hunger in Ireland, *see* Keys, *op. cit.,* p. 1251.
53. Patten, John: *English Towns: 1500-1700.* London, Dawson Archon Books, 1978, p. 135 (quoted from Flinn, M.W.: The stabilization of mortality in pre-industrial western Europe. *Journal of European History, 3*:285, 1974.
54. Fourastié, 1960, *op. cit.,* p. 69.
55. *Ibid,* p. 70.
56. *Ibid,* p. 71.

57. *Ibid.*, p. 74.
58. *Encyclopedia Britannica*, Vol. 4. Chicago, 1971, p. 787 ff.
59. de Castro, Josué: *The Black Book of Hunger*, translated by Charles L. Markmann. New York, Funk and Wagnalls, 1967, p. 7; the following figures are also taken from de Castro.
60. *Ibid.*, p. 10.
61. *Ibid.*, p. 10.
62. Hickey, Tom: *Health and Aging*. Monterey, Calif., Brooks/Cole Pub. Co., 1980.
63. McKeown, Thomas and Brown, R.G.: Medical evidence related to English population changes in the eighteenth century, in Glass, D.V. and Eversley, D.E.C.: *Population in History*. London, Edw. Arnold, 1965, p. 291; McKeown, Thomas: *The Modern Rise of Population*. New York, Academic Press, 1976, pp. 91-109.
64. Dubos, René: *Mirage of Health*. New York, Doubleday, 1961, p. 129.
65. George, M. Dorothy: *London Life in the 18th Century*. New York, Capricorn Books, 1965, pp. 50-51.
66. *Ibid.*, p. 32.
67. Akerknect, Erwin H.: *A Short History of Medicine*. New York, Ronald Co., 1955, p. 195; this, of course, refers to rates rather than absolute numbers.
68. Dubos, *op. cit.*, p. 204.
69. Akerknect, *op. cit.*, p. 196.
70. Diarrheal diseases were defined as diarrhea, dysentry, enteritis, cholera mobus, and cholera infantum by the U.S. census of 1880.
71. Farber, Harold K. and McIntosh, Rustin: *The History of the American Pediatric Society, 1887-1965*. New York, McGraw-Hill, 1966, p. 4-5.
72. *Ibid.*, p. 171.
73. Coale, Ansley J.: How a population ages or grows younger. In Friedman, Ronald: *Population: The Vital Revolution*. Chicago, Aldine, 1964, p. 51.
74. Subcommittee on Human Services of the Select Committee on Aging, U.S. House of Representatives: *Future Directions for Aging Policy: A Human Service Model*. Washington, D.C., U.S. Government Printing Office. No. 96-226, 1980, p. 99.
75. Preston, Samuel H.: *Mortality Patterns in National Populations: With Special Reference to Recorded Causes of Death*. New York, Academic Press, 1976, p. 57.
76. Sauvy, Alfred: *Fertility and Survival*. New York, Criterion Books, 1961, pp. 40-41.
77. Jacobson, *op. cit.*, p. 49.
78. Personal letter from Paul H. Jacobson (November 23, 1981).

Chapter 3

LONGEVITY AND LIFE PERSPECTIVE

TIME and timing are essential elements in a discussion of longevity and its social consequences. The dimensions of time give reality to the prospect of change, as well as to change itself. Few time periods are as important as those that pertain to length of life. There is a close connection between the awareness of time as finite, a serious interest in its measurement, and industrialization. The prolongation of life developed simultaneously with the cluster of cultural phenomena surrounding the rise of technology and industry. In modern society, both "time and treasure present themselves . . . . insistently as scarce and valuable elements in the basic problems of human existence."

In fact, "time with us (Americans) is handled much like material; we earn it, spend it, save it, waste it."[1] "As a rule, Americans think of time as a road or a ribbon stretching into the future, along which one progresses."[2] As a leading industrial society, Americans are expected to be almost completely future oriented. Conceptions of time, however, vary greatly from one culture to another. Native North Americans, such as people of the Pueblo and the Navajo, view the modern industrialized conceptions of time as foreign and inapplicable. To the Algerian peasant, "time stretches out, given a rhythm by the round of work and holidays and by the succession of nights and days. Time so marked is not . . . ., measured time. The intervals of subjective experience are not equal and uniform. The effective points of reference in the continued flux of time's passage are qualitative nuances read upon the surface of things."[3]

Life ordered by specific units, which are based on the Newtonian theory of time, are not, apparently, closely correlated with any rhythmic biological characteristics of man. It has been estimated by authorities on child development that the average child in the United States learns the basic technical workings of time by the age of twelve approximately, but takes much longer to master the social importance and emotional connotations of time.[4]

It seems appropriate that this exploration of the consequences of long life is occurring at a point in history, when treasure has apparently become so plentiful that a whole society can be defined as affluent.[5] Conceivably, further exploration will turn to our affluence of time.[6] In a broad sense, the history of our conception of time is one that takes us, basically, from vague and relatively lengthy units to minute and precise measures of time. Contrary to logic, "time scarcity in some absolute sense may be greatest where man's relations with his environment are extremely insecure as the ordinary state of affairs. Thus many nonliterate or 'primitive' groups have poorly developed techniques for providing sustenance and for the preservation of individual lives. Yet the uncertainty of life generally does not produce a careful fractionation of temporal units, a tidy husbanding of the 'manifestly' short and precarious supply."[7]

Moore refers to the paradox of people gaining actual living time, but perceiving time as being more scarce. He contends that two characteristics of modern civilization account for this: (1) the extreme specialization of and variety in social roles, and (2) the development of a means for precise measurement of time. Another important factor should be added, that being the steady increase in secularization and rationality and the concomitant decline in the sacred and supernatural. In elaborating on the paradox, Moore used the term "discretionary time." With the prolongation of life and freedom from a constant concern with subsistence, man has more time to use at his own discretion. A new kind of freedom has been added to the human condition. Despite this added increment of time, the perception of the scarcity of time persists. The frequent laments about "the awful rush," "the rat race," and the common excuse that "I don't have time," characterize the lives of those with the greatest amount of discretionary living time.

It seems apparent that the foregoing paradoxes pertaining to perceived scarcity of time are the result of a perspective of life that has emerged with longevity and the many other changes brought about by modern, urban, industrial society. This new perspective is one that includes a strong orientation towards a future in which man will be free from the more compelling vagaries of the natural world such as premature death from starvation, disease, or wild animals.

Although the empirical possibility of a life free from imminent death is recent, the conception and desire for such a life is ancient. An early Sumerian tablet (circa 5000 B.C) refers to the vision of a "Golden Age" when no snakes, scorpions, lions, hyenas, wild dogs, or wolves struck fear and terror in the hearts of men. It was a time when men had many rivals, and the future was always tentative. Though modern man has few natural rivals and death is no longer imminent, he must live with other terrors brought about by himself.

Longevity and Life Perspective

It seems plausible that an extended lifetime will transform a person's view of life, whether or not he or she is fully aware of the specific facts about life expectancy and longevity. Social scientific logic seems to require that the frequency of the death experience will have an impact on a person's life perspective. The probability that at least half of one's children will die young, that mothers frequently die in childbirth, and that we may not live more than a decade after midlife, are all contributory influences in affecting perspective. Similarities in the personal histories of people provide the raw material from which life perspectives are drawn. Death is one of the paramount features in shaping the lives of people and the way in which they perceive their lives. Death always leaves a gap in the social network in which each individual has played a part.

A close and constant familiarity with death has characterized the lives of people throughout most of human history. The experience of death has been augmented by many cultural practices or folkways, even some that deliberately court death for the young. We can speculate about the view of life that allowed the male to exercise the bravado and disdain for death that is associated with jousting, dueling, and individualized combat in warfare. What kind of life perspective was current in 1804 when the forty-nine year old Alexander Hamilton was legally killed in a duel with Aaron Burr? Hamilton's son, Philip, had been killed in a duel three years earlier. In the past and even now, manliness in western societies has demanded a certain amount of bravado and flirting with death. During times of relatively short life, a disdain for death may not have appeared as foolhardy as it does now, when a mature person can fully expect to live well past seventy.

The frequent experience of death among those close to one and uncertainty regarding the fatality of disease or accident are reflected in man's conception of the past, present, and future. In fact "no act of man is possible with reference solely to the past or solely to the future, but is always dependent on their interaction. Thus for example, the future may be considered as the horizon against which plans are made, the past provides the means for their realization, while the present mediates and actualizes both."[8] Thus, the living time available to the individual, based on knowledge of life expectancy in the past and the frequency of premature death in the present, gives some shape and substance as to how one should treat the present, as well as the feasibility of planning for the future. One's significant interpersonal relations, with kin group, family, and friends, are a critical aspect of that here and now.

No social research provides evidence for asserting or not that the present day remoteness of death in everyday life has an influence on the types of social relations characterized as violent and inhuman, or that the change in the timing of death meant an increase in the frequency of humane and affectionate relationships. But the frequency and timing of death among the various groups in society might well have a bearing on future answers. The fact that modern society is the scene of considerable interpersonal conflict that results in hatred and personal destruction does not necessarily mean that the relative absence of death (until old age) is of little consequence. This is especially true since the prolongation of life is a recent occurrence in human history. It is conceivable that we are only beginning to respond to a relatively long life, free from the age-old uncertainty of imminent death. Some of the recent revulsion toward death and destruction caused by the war in Indo-China may be related to an emerging perspective of life that makes death only legitimate when it occurs in old age or from incurable disease.

The almost total disappearance of public hangings, guillotining, and flogging conveys the impression that a change in public sensibilities may have taken place. The controversy over the use of capital punishment in the western world has led to a curious anomaly. In 1971, there were over 600 men officially awaiting execution in the United States, there having been no executions during the previous four years. The first execution to take place after the long moratorium occurred in January, 1977.

Repelled by the savage crowds he saw at the public hangings in Newgate prison yard, Charles Dickens concluded that the primary effect of official killings was to brutalize the public. It is possible that the emerging social awareness of the fact that acts against individuals can affect the body politic in a negative way is becoming more widespread. The conception that socially sanctioned brutality can harm society and those who are victims of capital punishment is certainly not a new idea, though its inclusion in the general social consciousness may be.

The full development and diffusion of ideas, however, is closely related to the social and cultural milieu in which they first emerge. For most of human history, these milieux have been strongly influenced by a close proximity to death. Recorded history provides little information on the everyday lives, values, attitudes, and expectations of the ordinary members of the human community. Therefore, it is difficult to determine the exact effects of variation in the timing of death through historical time.

During any short period of history, death rates appear to operate quite consistently across age levels. Therefore, people pay little attention to variation in these rates. Death is also frequently considered to be the great leveler. It is thought to affect all people somewhat evenly. The general assumption is that a person's length of life and one's objective condition of life are relative from one generation to the next. To a certain degree, this assumption is not fully adequate. It is adequate in that the basic recurring events in the lives of individuals and their families seem quite familiar from one generation or cohort to the next. This means, that extensive demographic changes, over time, are not consciously perceived and considered in the ordering of everyday behavior. That is, the full effect of the decline in premature death has not been fully discerned. The tacit assumption of relativity regarding the effect of a changing pattern in the timing of death is inadequate, because irrespective of the level of awareness that exists regarding a specific set of life conditions, the actual objective changes may have profound effects. The objective transformations with which we are concerned are those resulting from the recent shift in the timing of death. The implications of this change are broad. For example, the radical declines in infant, maternal, young adult, and middle-aged death represent important modifications.

W.R. Bytheway has written one of the few technical papers on the social consequences of death in a specific population. Using Scottish demographic data for 1966, he simulated the number and timing of deaths that a male would have experienced among his acquaintances and spouses as he aged from fifty to eighty years.[9] The simulation was based on the Scottish age-specific death rates at the time. Bytheway's paper was directed towards drawing inferences about possible relationships between the probability of death and chronological age; as such, his study appears distinctly original. The author's rationale for the importance of his study is the same as that which supports this work.

Bytheway cogently relates age, death, and peer group influences in his discussion. He quotes Loether: "The possibility of one's own death is most likely to enter awareness when one's relatives or friends die. Particularly when acquaintances of one's own age die, one is likely to be thinking about death in more personal terms."[10] Bytheway points out that when an aging man perceives that his peer acquaintances have not died prematurely as a result of accidents, but "of their own accord," that is, "as a result of reaching the 'rational' end of their lives," one "begins to see death as normative behavior for his age-group. The deceased are no longer parties to deviant acts. The deceased have behaved appropriately for their age. Deaths of his friends may have a certain poignancy. He attends their funerals, but these are anticipated (if random) events that become part of his regulated life, like visits from his adult children, and wins on the horses."[11]

Death as normative behavior is a key dimension of life that could only emerge with a certain level of longevity and a decrease in the capriciousness of death. Throughout human existence, most men and women did not die "natural" deaths. Death for almost everyone, more or less, was a deviant act. Under such circumstances, overall life perspective must have been considerably different from what it may become under circumstances of long life. As large numbers of people live longer and when death becomes defined as appropriate for one's peers as well as oneself, a new life perspective will have emerged. When death becomes "normal" in the latter stages of life, one's self-conception takes on new social psychological dimensions. They are dimensions that alter and change as one proceeds through a long and potentially varied life course. These critical social psychological changes in the lives of a great number of people must, of necessity, have an influence on society.

One of the notable characteristics of human beings is their capacity to adapt, and death is one of the critical events toward which this capacity must be directed. Unfortunately, the lack of historical data on the life of ordinary people in the past hinders the social investigation of adaptation to a high prevalence of death. What social scientific evidence we have is from extreme conditions involving the spectre of imminent premature death in recent times, and it is generally psychological rather than sociological in perspective. Furthermore, the literature of the past provides us, primarily, with examples of special situations involving the experience of death.

Social and Psychic Responses to Frequent Death

Though scanty, there is some evidence from the concentration camp experience and from the bombing of Hiroshima during World War II that imminent death and deprivation have serious effects on the social psychological functioning of those who are involved. Both Kogon and Lifton refer to "dulled sensibilities" or "psychic numbing" resulting from the intense experience of death, horror, pain, and grief that characterized life in the German concentration camps and the postbomb period of Hiroshima.[12] Although life in past centuries cannot be deemed comparable to the horrendous conditions existent during World War II, the imminence of death and the uncertainty surrounding life for the millions who experienced the Black Death, famine, flood, cholera, and countless diseases must have created somewhat similar psychological consequences.

The chroniclers of disasters like those of the Black Death or of famines and epidemics, emphasize extremes in social behavior. A common response to death's omnipresence was to "eat, drink and be merry, for tomorrow we may die."[13] It was reported that London, during the Plague, was the scene of "drinking, roaring and surfeiting. . . . In one house you might hear them roaring under the pangs of death, in the next tippling, whoring and belching out blasphemies against God."[14]

Those who were believed to have contracted one of the devastating diseases of the period suffered a social death. Persons with whom each individual had been socially linked through kinship, friendship, or business made every effort to avoid them. Sorokin comments on the social and psychological consequences of calamities like plague: "The victim is in the position of a spider whose web has been torn asunder. The former subject — or active participant in social life — is turned into a helpless object, avoided, forsaken, and repellent. He ceases to form a part of society. Socially he is already dead though he is still alive biologically."[15]

Perhaps the most common response to the abhorrent conditions of earlier life was an extravagant religiosity. "The pestilence was almost universally regarded . . . as the manifestation of the wrath of an aroused God punishing mankind for its wickedness."[16] Many people gave the Church gifts and made extravagant pledges and vows to change future behavior. Conduct veered from an extreme of license and debauchery to piety and financial commitments to the church. The uncertainty of life bred extreme and erratic behavior.

Violence and crime accompanied the disasters of the plague. "Burial gangs looted the houses of the dead and stripped the corpses of anything of value . . . On occasion they even murdered the sick."[17] Others, thinking themselves moral and pious, accused and hunted witches or anyone else that might be blamed for bringing the plague by supernatural or natural means. John Calvin believed that witches were responsible for introducing the plague to Geneva. It is possible that the righteous had to have a scapegoat. God's wrath in the form of disaster and pestilence would otherwise have been inexplicable. For the Calvinist, the presence of the plague in Geneva, God's city, would seem otherwise imcomprehensible.

The epidemics, famines, and disasters that often made life a living hell were not an everyday phenomena, even in the distant past. Nevertheless, the frequency of famines and epidemics made them all too commonplace to avoid the conclusion that they were an important part of life for a great many people. The fluctuations in the price of grain often made "ordinary" hunger an annual affair during certain periods in the history of Europe.[18] There seems to be little doubt that the prevalence of death and its uncertainties had a profound influence on those aspects of human life that shaped the view that people had of life itself.

At the end of the period (nineteenth century) of high mortality from infectious diseases such as tuberculosis, the prospects of early death evoked sentimentality. Alexandre Dumas wrote in his memoirs

(1823-24), ". . . it was the fashion to suffer from the lungs; everybody was consumptive, poets especially; it was good form to spit blood after each emotion that was at all sensational, and to die before reaching the age of thirty."[19] By the end of the nineteenth century such a sentimental fashion was becoming outmoded, and was probably confined to a relatively small segment of the population, although it was a culturally important minority. For the rank and file of mankind, the dangers leading to death evoked a fear that was dealt with, primarily, by a great variety of myths, magic rituals, and religion. Since the fears and terrors of premature death have generated a vast amount of myth and ritual, any change in the timing or incidence of death will have important social psychological consequences.

Famine also contributed to premature death and had important social psychological effects. Famine and starvation are not only painful but lead to certain extremes in psychological functions. "Apathy, quickly replaced by irritability is . . . . uniformly noted by most of the observers or self observers of starvation in actual life."[20] "Dull and hopeless apathy was the main characteristic of the masses in the famine years of the Middle Ages."[21] The same has been said for the later famines in China, Russia, and India.

Life Expectancy and Secular Perspective

Secularization, which concerns many of those who value the metaphysical and religious aspects of life, functions as both cause and effect in analyzing the change in life perspective. Secularization may have resulted from the fact that longevity has contributed to a more rational response to death. The centuries of human experience involving reactions to sudden and unanticipated death contributed to a sense of mystery and speculation about the unknown. Death, in most cases, is no longer cloaked in mystery. By the ability to postpone deaths at almost all ages along the life span, medical science has done much to promote a more secular interpretation of both life and death.

A high mortality rate and short life expectancy would enhance the aspect of religion that concerns itself with life after death. The decline of premature death may partially explain why religious organizations have had to reorient their approach in order to maintain their membership. The importance of a belief in life after death, or the transmigration of souls, has declined in the industrialized countries. The change in the timing of death has altered our conception of life. In modern industrial society, the role of religious organizations in connection with death seem to be primarily ritualistic. They serve the function of formalizing and ritualizing the passage from life to death. This is essentially true for deaths that are not premature in that they occur in old age. In effect, longevity has legitimized death, and as such, the needs for an afterlife have seemingly declined. In fact, social science, as a specific development in the overall rise of science, appears to be providing some kind of substitute for various features of traditional religion. Social knowledge helps one to cope with the vicissitudes of life and diminishes the necessity of looking to an afterlife for relief from frustrations and troubles that arise. This has furthered the development of a rhetoric of rationality in the solving of human problems.

The demand for social scientific knowledge has been stimulated by the fact that longevity has thrust a new set of social problems into focus. This is true for the problems that beset people whose lives are prolonged until they retire or who live on and on without an adequate place in the social scheme with all manner of physical and economic disabilities. The scientific skills in maintaining life have reached such extremes that serious questions have arisen as to the appropriateness of keeping people alive when the hope of recovery to any satisfactory state of health is questionable. Some articulate old people have voiced the desire for a dignified death, free from the impersonal and frightening prelude to dying that characterizes the mechanical and chemical artificiality of the intensive care units of modern hospitals.

A highly rational societal response to the problems of death faced by some cancer victims is seen in an organization called Cancer Care.[22] This organization is an arm of the National Cancer Foundation. It has served thousands of families and spent millions providing social services to individuals and families who were faced with a death from cancer. Such social organizations have done much to promote a rational approach to death.

The lessening of death's disruptiveness has had an effect on many human activities in which the use of rational thought is characteristic. As religion has lost ground, education and science have gained. Rational approaches have pushed these activities to great lengths.

Future Orientation and Longevity

Of the three dimensions of time, past, present, and future, the future has been most vitally affected by longevity. To most people prior to modern times, the future was very precarious and uncertain. The preindustrial Algerian peasant, who represents an age-old social type, was governed chiefly by traditions and the rhythms of everyday life. Time was not something that one made plans for, aggressively used, or saved. The peasant's conception of the future was dim and planless. Such a perspective had decided effects on daily life and thought, but planning, individual achievement, or investment for future gains were not among them. Fear was the characteristic reaction to time and life.

Feuer states that traditional societies are characterized by a fatalistic spirit "common to all peasant societies, whether Egyptian, Mexican, or Indonesian, which have seen an eternal sameness in things, with the defeat of every rising generation predestined." The Egyptian fellah who lives "always under fear, his entire social life . . . controlled by endemic fear, despising his work and his life, rooted to the ground, is typical of the human foundation of traditional society."[23] One of the profound changes accompanying the age revolution is the development of future orientation on the part of many in modern industrial society.

Though many societies of the world are now experiencing greater longevity than ever, they have not fully recognized the possibilities offered by the prolongation of life. There is, moreover, a difference between perceiving or realizing that one has a relatively long life ahead and actively planning for that future. Planning can take place at all stages of the life course. Though little research has dealt with future orientation in the context presented here, there are studies that reveal the complexity of the problem and the difficulty of assessing the factors responsible for generating a future orientation. One study of young people reveals the variations found in the relationship between goals or desires and plans made to implement the goals. This study attempted to assess the future ambitions of beginning students (ninth grade) in several American high schools:

Stephenson found that although there was relatively little variation regarding ambitions between students from different social strata, there were substantial differences in the plans for achieving stated ambitions.[24] A large proportion of the students wanted to become high status professionals like doctors, lawyers, engineers, and so on. A relatively small proportion, however, had made definite plans for higher education and were acting in a manner consistent with the achievement of these goals. The majority of those who had made realistic plans and were following them were in the middle and upper social strata.

Fraisse found that workingmen generally refused to imagine the possibility of a long period of study or training for either themselves or their children.[25] A common response was "that isn't for us." It was also observed that the frequency of payment for work had an effect on temporal orientation. Wage workers who are paid by the week or in some instances by the day have a different perspective than persons who are on an annual salary and are paid by the month. The latter mode of payment demands considerably greater planning and stimulates a larger horizon than does the weekly paycheck.

There is no doubt that one's view of the future, or the realistic evaluation of imagined possibilities for the life ahead, has something to do with objective factors in the individual's personal situation. "Planning cannot *in practice* overstep the horizon of the possible."[26] Power, wealth, family background, long life, and relative freedom from some of the uncertainties surrounding high rates of premature death are pertinent to the kind of future orientation that is possible for the various segments of a given society.

An example of how a dramatic change in circumstances can change old habits and facilitate a new future-oriented perspective of life is recounted by Bourdieu. In 1954, a factory in Algeria raised its wages by 20 percent. The logic of the workers dictated that they should only work enough to provide the income necessary to meet their customary demands. Therefore, the large raise in wages led to a 20 percent reduction in the hours that they were willing to work. In fact, they seemed to prefer the free time over extra wages. Factory managers raised wages again, this time doubling them, which amounted to a 240 percent raise over the initial wage. Bourdieu observed the following: "The consequences of this second increase were radically different from those of the first. As if a threshold had been broken, the workers showed a desire to work, to earn even more, to work overtime, to anticipate the future by thrift. It was as if the whole of their attitude toward the world had undergone a complete restructuring as a result of the modification of a single trait, as if, freed from his anxiety over subsistence, the individual suddenly discovered that he was capable of taking his own future in is hands."[27] The change in the economic situation of the tradition-oriented Algerian took place on a scale so great that it was impossible for the worker not to perceive that a shift in work habits could transform his life chances so drastically; rapid social change ensued.

In contrast to the immediacy of the consequences that are brought on by a sudden change in economic circumstances, the ramifications of the control of death and longevity will be discovered slowly and will probably not be as dramatic. Unfortunately, few if any studies have been done relating life perspective or future orientation to longevity. The difficulty in studying the consequences of longevity in terms of life perspective is primarily due to the lack of available information about the everyday life of the common man in the past and present. Even when the information is at hand in the present, little or nothing has been reported on the social psychological consequences of the great decline in mortality rates, as in Ceylon following the introduction of DDT and modern drugs.[28]

The great change in the chronology of life resulting from the gradual decline in death rates and increased longevity has not provided the kind of vivid social changes that are discernible, for example, in the doubling of income by the Algerian peasants. Also, the finality and inevitablity of death has given it an entirely different meaning from that attached to income or wealth.

It takes more than a general change in the conditions of modern life, such as longevity, to explain the emergence of new temporal perspectives. Comparing two different occupational groups, two social scientists showed that time perspective may be greatly affected by relationships between the current work mode and the history of groups. Benard and Blanchard studied a Norman village comprised of two very different populations, an historical group of farmers (peasants) and a new group of laborers in a glass works. The two groups exhibited vastly different temporal perspectives:

The peasants, rooted in their soil, have a large temporal horizon oriented toward the past; the history of their families has been that of their lands and their buildings. They have also constructed a spacious future: plans for buying land, for building, for getting their children established.

The glassworkers, on the other hand, are a group of immigrants coming, for the most part, from Brittany. Cut off as they are from their origins and their familial ties, the past has little reality for them; their future, with little prospect of promotion, is also very constricted. They live confronted only by immediate problems, and even the future of their children seems to them a mere prolongation of their routine existence.[29]

It is apparent that the future orientation of the Norman peasants was, partially, a function of the fact that they owned their land, could accumulate capital, and had a history of some minimal kind of achievement in the course of their lives. They cannot be counted as peasants of the variety that occupied the world from the beginning of agriculture to the industrial revolution. They are, in a sense, modern farmers. The demands of their occupation and its apparent potentialities have stimulated an orientation towards a future. In contrast, the glass-workers have a social and occupational history that breeds a very similar perspective to that of the Algerian peasant; one that is fatalistic and traditional.

Future Orientation and Achievement

It is difficult to develop an effective conception of achievement in a social context in which the primary emphasis is on the present. Speculation and planning for the future is inhibitied in such a social context. The tradition-bound peasant, for example, is closely limited to the actions and thoughts of everyday life. The development and use of rational calculation is frequently repressed in traditional society. The Algerian peasant does not count the number of chickens hatched, the number of men at a meeting, nor determine the amount of seed grain one has set aside for planting. Such acts are presumptuous, for "the future belongs to God," which means that it can in no way, belong to man.[30] These kinds of proscriptions prevent the development of the view that the future is a time for realizing possibilities, and that there may be a chance that something new, different, or even better might take place. A future orientation demands the opening of one's life to chance and the possibility that something unforeseen may occur. According to Parsons, "The projection of the possible is the basis of every belief in progress."[31]

As Parsons implies, achievement demands a future. One question that poses itself is, how is the prolongation of life related to one's view of the future? Since few young men can seriously believe that they will ever die, we must assume that the young have a great potential for adopting an orientation that includes projection and planning. Some psychologists, among them Henry A. Murray, have attempted to deal with the question of how one's future perspective is altered by the prospect of longevity. Murray has hypothesized that man is characterized by *ascensionism*, which may be defined in the following:

> . . . as an integrate of the need for achievement and a relatively much stronger need for awed attention, for spectacular glory, for sensational prestige, which may or may not be linked with a component of sexuality, the special aim of this compound being to ascend vertically, in a physical, social, or intellectual sense. . . . In primitive religions, particularly in Greek mythology, there were scores of gods, demigods, and heroes who ascended to high places — the summit of Mt. Olympus, say, or some paradise in the upper regions of the sky. Here the goal was combined with imagined social ascensionism, since high places of this sort were occupied by the spiritual elite — aristocratic deities, choirs of angels, or a whole society of elected saints.[32]

In relating ascensionism to the American way of life, Murray suggests that prior to the American Revolution the desire for vertical achievement was confined, primarily, to a religious zeal that made entry into heaven the most desired achievement, despite the emergence of Puritanism and the Protestant Ethic. According to Murray, however, following the Revolution, the inherent human desire for achievement was secularized and translated into what may be characterized as the Horatio Alger myth, "the craving for upward social mobility by means of material success."[33]

Among some, short life expectancy might promote economic and status achievement for a life that might be short, but brilliant. Such a perspective might stimulate entrepeneurial fervor and personal aggrandizement. On the other hand, an awareness of long life would generate the kind of life perspective that measures achievement differently at various points or phases of the life course. What we do to achieve in one phase should be compatible with the plans and desires for later phases. At some points in the life course, achievement, as presently defined in competitive society, might be looked down upon and avoided.

According to Murray, although the young perceive themselves as indestructible and have an inherent drive to achieve, the contingencies relating to death and length of life have a bearing on how a future orientation will emerge. For example, at what point in the life course does one begin to entertain doubts about the future? Logically, the higher the death rate is among youth and young adults, the shorter the period there is in which to perceive oneself as having a future.[34] We have no adequate data on the rate at which one's age peers must die before a sense of fatality emerges and future orientation is inhibited.

A hypothesis can be advanced: the awareness of inevitable death in a society with relatively long duration of life occurs at the approximate midpoint of the expected length of life. At current death rates with an expected length of life of approximately seventy-two to seventy-six years, the midpoint comes at thirty-six to thirty-eight years of age.[35] It seems reasonable to assume that one's perspective of the future is affected by the midpoint in life. Calculations of this kind are, of course, only possible in societies that have precise ways of measuring time.

In line with the above hypothesis, one might argue that the five or so years after the midpoint of life could (or would) represent an important bench mark, though not always perceived as such. Scientific evidence supporting this is beginning to emerge from numerous studies in social gerontology done in Europe and the United States during the past decade.

One wonders how the ordinary man or woman could have developed the necessary attitudinal prerequisites for achievement when the average length of life was short. The vision of life as an ascending skyrocket may be a colorful way of describing a perception of a successful life, but it is applicable only to a small number of unique people. The idea of personal achievement as an important ingredient in the thoughtways of all individuals occurs after the Renaissance and is probably related to the control of death and prolongation of life. Throughout human history, some individuals have had a perspective that was oriented towards the future, although the present argument implies they were relatively few in number. In general, longevity is only one of the necessary prerequisites for the kind of future orientation that is associated with achievement. There are other social and psychological factors.

The possession of some kind of future orientation may have been limited by one's ascribed social roles or by one's individual characteristics, such as a special talent. The latter, of course, would have to manifest itself early in one's life. In past ages, there was no time for the slow learner or late bloomer. Those social roles that placed the individual in a position wherein he or she could be effective in carrying out a change in the condition of life allowed the individual to develop a future orientation. Only those who achieved great leadership position, power, or wealth would have the resources needed to seriously plan for the future. It is apparent that the upper strata in medieval and renaissance Europe enjoyed a greater longevity than the common people, though the advantage was not very large at times and had no great bearing on overall life-expectancy during times of epidemic and pandemic diseases.[36]

People in the modern industrial countries who concern themselves with a wide range of social, political, and economic problems can do so with relatively little concern about the risk of death from common illnesses until late middle or old age. At sixty years of age, contemporary men and women can avoid some of the stigma of old age, as well as the fear of imminent and premature death. Despite the long life expectancy reported in demographic statistics, premature deaths do occur with greater frequency as each birth cohort advances in years. In spite of the prospect of long life, some people have difficulty in coming to terms with the process of growing older. As a consequence, they view a great part of their lives in a fatalistic manner, similar to our peasant ancestors.

The issue of fertility and birth control is linked to life perspective. Referring to the earlier discussion of the Algerian peasants' view of time, we find that in order to accept birth control, a recognition of the efficiency of rational planning is necessary. If we do not accept the possibility of rational planning, we submit to natural fertility, in addition to all of the other submissions to nature, fate, the gods, and so on. Life becomes what Bourdieu calls traditionalistic. Changing from the traditionalistic perspective to the "calculating and predictive" attitude, the individual must view himself or herself as being in conflict with nature. Changing to this viewpoint and ceasing to submit to the given of nature, we have taken on "the goal of another possible world which can come into existence only by the transformation of the present state of the world."[37] Moreover, "some evidence exists . . . to support the view that fertility varies with what has been called 'the future time perspective' of individuals and that this perspective varies from occupation to occupation, possibly because of the nature of the relationship between an individual's work (thought of as life chance) and the time factor."[38]

Beshers has categorized three different "modes of orientation" that have varying affects on the decision- making process involved in birth control: traditional, short-run hedonistic, and purposive-rational modes. Beshers states the following:

> From a decision viewpoint a crucial difference among the modes of orientation is the future time perspective. The traditional mode of orientation implies no crystalized future time perspective for an individual. There is no sequential decision making. The individual acting in the traditional mode selects the same alternative that he selected before with no recourse to new information. He follows custom. . . The individual acting in the short-run hedonistic mode has a very brief future time perspective. The calculation of likelihoods and of utilities takes account of a brief time period in the future. . . The individual acting in the purposive-rational mode has an elaborate time perspective extending far into the future. His calculation of likelihoods and of utilities is complex and intricate, and is very sensitive to new information.[39]

The problem of assessing whether or not a particular combination of behaviors fall into the short-run hedonist or the purposive-rational mode is illustrated by the following comparison. A recent cross-cultural comparison of orientations toward the future appears to show important differences between older persons in Poland and America. ". . . That older Americans, like other Americans, are content to live for the present, to 'fly now and pay later,' in the words of a popular advertisement. To live just for the day is apparently not an accepted mode of behavior in Polish life. The future cannot be allowed to take care of itself. It must be planned. This kind of emphasis on future planning is perhaps a result of the important role that agriculture played for so long in the Polish economy. No farmer could prosper if he lived 'just for today.' "[40] It is implied that the Polish farmer is more future oriented than the American farmer. In some sense this may be true, but an important consideration has been overlooked in making this kind of generalization. The very possibility of having personal credit that allows the American to fly now and pay later presumes that the debtor will probably live long enough to pay it back, or will be protected by a life insurance policy to cover his indebtedness if he were to die prematurely. The price and practicality of that policy will have been determined by known life expectancy rates. The variations in orientation, implied by Shanas, are based on the assumption that the way in which social groups view their future is determined by the culture of which they are a part. In some instances, occupation may be more relevant than in others. The Poles manifest purposive-rational behavior, which is also true for the elderly retired American. The Americans based their behavior on an intricate financial and legal system of the most advanced purposive-rational type — even though the manifest behavior, reported by Shanas, seems to be of the short-run hedonistic kind. The signing of credit papers in the airline office has brought forth considerable rational calculation, as to the future prospects for paying the ensuing monthly charges. If this were not the case, the massive credit system of the United States would have collapsed long ago. This indicates the care needed in the analysis of time perspectives attributed to various types of social categories or groups. In effect, both aged Polish farmers and American retirees, are behaving rationally, and the hedonistic label seems misplaced.

It is possible that deliberate, rational planning and calculations of all types relating to the future may decrease as certain types of social organizations take over the planning function. On the level of personal planning and calculation, modern society has provided a layer of assurances for the future by the development of nondiscretionary systems of saving. Life insurance, old age annuity plans (government pension and social security systems) and house mortgage payments are illustrative. These involve an initial period of rational planning activity, after which the costs are treated as recurring financial obligations. This approach is an important aspect in the development of programs and concepts, such as unemployment insurance, guaranteed minimum incomes, guaranteed annual income, old age pension systems, and medical insurance.

Thus, despite the increasing length of life, many of the features of life that have demanded foresight and planning, are removed from the control of the individual citizen. This might allow individuals to spend more time planning their future in matters not directly related to the problems of subsistence or the consumption of surplus wealth. Instead, aspects of life involving human pleasure and personal development could be wholeheartedly pursued.

One of the salient features of the life perspective that emerged with the break-up of feudalism was the future orientation that accompanied the Protestant Ethic. This developed powerful social motivations toward hard work. Work became virtually sanctified. According to Weber, this was an ethic that was accompained by a religious conviction that the safest way to insure election to a good afterlife was through productive work — a Calvininst invention.[41]

In this context, it must not be forgotten that the devout Puritans of New England were not only major proponent of the Protestant Ethic, but also deeply preoccupied with death. This was true despite the fact that they were not subject to inordinantly high death rates; they were healthier and lived longer than their relatives in England. This is an example of their thinking: ". . . it was the unquestioned duty of every right-thinking Puritan to keep the thought of death ever on his mind. . . Even children were early immersed in the required preoccupation of their elders, whether learning the alphabet and encountering such rhymes as: 'G — As runs the *Glass*/Man's life does pass;/T — *Time* cuts down all/Both great and small;/X — *Xerxes* the great did die/And so must you & I;/Y — *Youth* forward slips/Death soonest nips.' "[42] Despite the intense fear of death experienced by the early New Englanders, their acceptance of the Protestant ethic of work makes sense because work and its fruits were viewed as a positive sign — one that signified consignment to heaven rather than to hell. Stannard points out that their great fear of death was based on a belief in their own depravity. They believed in God's preeminent power and justness and the indescribable horrors of hell.[44] The thought of death stimulated an orientation that looked toward a future leading to heaven while simultaneously utilizing time on earth in a manner that was achievement oriented with respect to worldly matters. Although modern times have seen a radical decline in the Puritan fear of death, the ethic of work was perpetuated through child-rearing practices and became an integral part of the definition of adult social roles in large parts of Europe and the new world.

In contrast, a study of the psychological consequences of concern about death on the time perspective of college-aged youth indicates that those who are concerned or preoccupied with death seem "to live more in the present than in the future."[44] Among modern youth, concerns about death may not be conditioned by Puritan attitudes.

Spread of the Protestant Ethic throughout Europe is yet to be fully documented; however, as illustrated by the limited and routine experience of glass-workers referred to earlier, it is apparent that the social and occupational history of a specific family or group can create a life perspective that appears almost futureless. The same can be said of the thousands of contemporary urban poor, who can see little beyond survival from one day to the next. A recent study reports that the contemporary hard core poor have a conception of time comparable to that of the aforementioned Algerian peasant; ". . . . to the hard core poor, time is a series of discrete moments, each understood in itself rather than a continuum."[45] Conceptions like social mobility, infinity, and the relative value of money are generally not an important part of the cognitive characteristics of the long-term poor. Though such a perception of time may be deeply rooted in language itself, it is also a result of the long-term deprivation characterizing the everyday lives of the urban poor. Conjoined with the usual forms of deprivation are the relatively high rates of disease, debilitation, and death among both the urban poor and Algerian peasants.[46]

Though Max Weber related the Protestant Ethic to the "spirit of capitalism," it is obvious that life and work under traditional capitalism, may do more to inhibit than enhance an orientation toward achievement and a better future for many of those at the lower end of the stratification scale.

A perspective that promotes the importance of work and efficiency is closely connected to achievement and orientation to the future. If the precariousness of life makes achievement difficult to envision or plan for, it is difficult to assume that zeal toward work could be assigned a positive value. The development of an orientation toward future achievement may have been concomitant with the emergence of the work ethic. In order that work be valued, it had to pay off in some way or another. Although the Calvinist may have been working for a future life in heaven, the majority of those who adopted the work ethic, in the Western World, were not Calvinists, and many in the United States were not Protestants; for them, the rewards of work had to be more tangible. This would depend on the assumption of avoiding an early death and a perspective free from the fatalism of traditional society.

With the modern development of strong cultural norms for encouraging individual achievement, the conditions for personal failure also emerged, as well as the recognition of it. Ariès states that "today the adult experiences sooner or later — and increasingly it is sooner — the feeling that he has failed, that his adult life has failed to achieve any of the promises of his adolescence. This feeling is at the basis of the climate of depression which is spreading throughout the leisured classes of industrialized societies."[47] This feeling, according to Ariès, was utterly foreign in the mental life of traditional societies. It began, however, to emerge among the powerful, rich, and learned men of the late Middle Ages:

> Nevertheless there is a very interesting difference between our contemporary feeling of personal failure and that found in the late Middle Ages. The certainty of death and the fragility of life are foreign to our existential pessimism. . . man of the late Middle Ages was very acutely conscious that he had merely been granted a stay of execution, that this delay would be a brief one and that death was always present within him, shattering his ambitions and poisoning his pleasure. And that man felt a love of life which we today can scarcely understand, perhaps because of our increased longevity.[48]

Long life has introduced a new dimension in the failures and vicissitudes of life. Advanced age means inevitable decline, both physically and socially. Important roles are lost, and those that are retained are emptied of much of their former content. This loss has been conceptualized as constituting a change from *institutional* roles to *tenuous* roles.[49] The diminished and half-empty tenuous roles characterize some of the major social losses of advanced age. Long life means that a large proportion of men and women will experience this new aspect of life. It is clearly apparent that the change in the timing of death has markedly influenced the norms, values, and expectations that develop at various points in the life course.

Long life, and its potential for effecting profound social consequences, is difficult to study; but despite the lack of direct measures of the effects of longevity, the thoughtways associated with future orientation and individuality warrant a continued search for more data, as well as new modes of analysis.

REFERENCES AND NOTES

1. Hall, Edward T.: *The Silent Language*. Garden City, New York, Doubleday, 1959, p. 29.

2. *Ibid.,* p. 28.
3. Bourdieu, Pierre: The attitude of the Algerian peasant toward time. In Pitt-Rivers, Julian (Ed.): *Mediterranean Countrymen.* Paris, Mouton and Co., 1963, p. 59.
4. Hall, *op. cit.,* p. 166.
5. Galbraith, John K.: *The Affluent Society.* Boston, Houghton Mifflin, 1958. The social implications of labeling American society as affluent has recently come under severe attack.
6. A recent book deals with time as a scarce value, a value that decreases as economic growth and general affluence increases. The affluence of time as a result of wealth seems mythical according to Linder, Staffan Burenstam: *The Harried Leisure Class.* New York, Columbia University Press, 1970.
7. Moore, Wilbert E.: *Man, Time, and Society.* New York, Wiley, 1963, p. 17.
8. Kummel, Friedrich: Time as succession and the problem of duration. In Fraser, J.T. (Ed.): *Voices of Time.* New York, George Braziller, 1966, p. 50.
9. Bytheway, W.R.: Aspects of old age in age-specific mortality rates. *Journal of Biosocial Science,* 2:337-349, 1970.
10. *Ibid.,* p. 338, quoted from Lowther, H.J.: *Problems of Aging.* Belmont, Calif., Dickenson Publishing Co., 1967.
11. *Ibid.,* p. 339.
12. Kogon, Eugene: *The Theory and Practice of Hell.* Translated by Heinz Norden, New York, Farrar, Straus Cudahy, 1951, p. 277; Lifton, Robert Jay: *Death in Life: Survivors of Hiroshima.* New York, Random House, 1967; Lifton, Robert Jay: *Boundaries: Psychological Man in Revolution.* New York: Simon and Schuster, 1969.
13. Langer, William: The black death, *Scientific American,* Feb., 1964, p. 117.
14. *Ibid.,* p. 117.
15. Sorokin, Pitrim: *Man and Society in Calamity.* New York, Dutton, 1942, p. 21.
16. Dubos, René J.: *Mirage of Health: Utopias, Progress, and Biological Change.* New York, Harper and Bros., 1959, p. 199.
17. Langer, *op. cit.,* p. 117.
18. Fourastié, Jean: *The Causes of Wealth.* Glencoe, Ill., The Free Press, 1960, pp. 59 ff.
19. Dubos, *op. cit.,* p. 206.
20. Sorokin, *op. cit.,* p. 18.
21. *Ibid.,* p. 19 quoted from Curshmann, F.: *Hungersmote in Mittelalter.* Leipzig, 1900, pp. 53 *et passim.*
22. *New York Times,* April 29, 1971, p. 50.
23. Feuer, Lewis S.: *The Conflict of Generations.* New York, Basic Books: 1969, p. 174.
24. Stephenson, Richard M.: Occupational aspirations and plans of 443 ninth graders. *Journal of Educational Research,* 49:27-35, 1955.
25. Fraisse, Paul: Of time and the worker. *Harvard Business Review,* 37:124, 1959.
26. *Ibid.,* p. 124.
27. Bourdieu, *op. cit.,* p. 71.
28. From 1945 to 1950 death rates for all age-groups exhibited a dramatic decline,

some dropping by as much as 65 percent. Department of Census and Statistics. *Statistical Abstract of Ceylon.* Colombo, Government Press, 1963, p. 61.

29. Quoted in Fraisse, Paul: Of time and the worker. *Harvard Business Review, 37*:124, 1959.

30. Bourdieu, *op. cit.,* p. 63.

31. Parsons, Talcott: Towards a healthy maturity. *Journal of Health and Human Behavior, 2*:163-174, 1960.

32. Murray, Henry H.: "Drive, time, strategy, measurement, and our way of life. In Lindzey, Gardner (Ed.): *Assessment of Human Motives.* New York, Rinehart, 1958, p. 193.

33. *Ibid.,* p. 194; Murray's analysis finds support from the fact that the phrase "getting ahead" does not seem to appear until 1807 and then again in 1951, *The Oxford English Dictionary,* Vol, IV, Oxford, Claredon Press, 1933, p. 142. Nevertheless, Murray's assumption that man possesses an inherent drive to achieve may be contested.

34. Moore, *op. cit.,* p. 54.

35. This midpoint will vary depending on whether life expectancy at birth or, for example, at 30 years is used. I trust the reader will forego the charge of misplaced precision in the above statistic — the figures are merely illustrative.

36. Antonovsky, Anton: Social class, life expectancy and overall mortality. *The Millbank Memorial Fund Quarterly, 45*:31-39, 1967; Peller, Sigismund: Births and deaths among Europe's ruling families since 1500. In Glass, D.V. and Eversley, D.E.C. (Eds.): *Population in History; Essays in Historical Demography.* London, Edward Arnold, 1965, pp. 87-100; Hollingsworth, T.H.: A demographic study of the British ducal families. *op. cit.,* pp. 354-378.

37. Bordieu, *op. cit.,* p. 71.

38. Banks, J.A.: Historical sociology and the study of population. *Daedalus, 97*:404, 1968; Banks attributes the "future time perspective" idea to Beshers, James M., *Population Processes in Social Systems.* New York, Free Press, 1967, p. 85.

39. Beshers, *op. cit.,* pp. 85-86.

40. Shanas, Ethel: Aging and life space in Poland and the United States. *Journal of Health and Social Behavior, 11*:185, 1970.

41. Weber, Max: *The Prostestant Ethic and the Spirit of Capitalism.* Trans. by Talcott Parsons, New York, Scribners, 1958.

42. Quoted from *The New England Primer.* 1727 facimile. New York, Paul Leicester Ford, 1962 in Stannard, David E.: Death and dying in puritan New England. *American Historical Review, 78* (December 1973), p. 1314.

43. Stannard, *op. cit.,* p. 1327.

44. Dickstein, Louis S. and Blatt, Sidney J.: Death concern futurity, and anticipation. *Journal of Consulting Psychology. 30*:15, 1966.

45. Cohen, Rosalie, Fraendel, Gerd and Brewer, John: The language of the hardcore poor: implications for culture conflict. *The Socio-logical Quarterly, 9*:25, 1968.

46. Since the poor may live relatively long lives, we cannot assert that longevity is a direct causal factor in emergence of a future orientation. We are only stating that factors such as high infant death rates and mobidity rates, have conse-

quence for attitudes toward the future.

47. Ariès, Phillipe: *Western Attitudes Toward Death: From the Middle Ages to the Present.* Trans. by Patricia M. Ranurn, Baltimore, Johns Hopkins University Press, 1974, p. 44.

48. *Ibid.*

49. Rosow, Irving: Status and role change through the life span. In Binstock, Robert H. and Shanas, Ethel: *Handbook of Aging and the Social Sciences.* New York, Van Nostrand Reinhold Co., 1976, pp. 462-80.

Chapter 4

PERSONAL CONSEQUENCES OF LONG LIFE

A S Chapters 2 and 3 indicate, long life has set the stage for a profound change in life perspective, the results of which are already being felt. One of the most important consequences of change in our social consciousness is how it affects the social and psychological aspects of individual lives. The effects of the change in the imminence of death and the emerging awareness of long life on youth, middle-aged, and elderly will be discussed. Consequences of long life will be explored in relation to the self-concept of those destined to live under modern conditions of longevity. Personal competence and self-control will be discussed, as well as social, psychological, and physiological losses incurred over a long life.

Long Life as It Affects Childhood, Youth, and Early Adulthood

The enormous change in the mortality rate of infants and children has consequences for both adults and children. A pervasive atmosphere of fear and destruction has been removed from the social consciousness of children. Children are no longer confronted with the necessity of coming to some kind of understanding regarding the death of brothers, sisters, or other age peers. Fear of the child's own death is greatly diminished for the modern child, though we have little scientific knowledge regarding this matter.

Change in the chronology of death has meant that children's fears of losing a parent through death has decreased. The orphanage is no longer an important institution, and childhood fears of being sent to an orphanage are almost unknown. A college class in sociology was recently asked if they knew of any orphanages in the city. Two students out of twenty answered in the affirmative. Our general affluence, development of social welfare, change in mortality rates, and life insurance contribute to a change in social consciousness.

The probability that a child will live to maturity and beyond has changed the way infants are perceived by adults. When children are no longer expected to die, parents can safely make a greater emotional investment in child rearing and parenthood. There is historical evidence that when a substantial proportion of infants and children were expected to die, everyone was psychologically prepared for the disaster of death. In seventeenth century France, infants that died were neither named or remembered as individuals.[1] The level of emotional involvement between parents and children had to be limited in order to preserve their sanity from the high probability of death. Such a restriction on emotional attachment and the resulting decrease in family intimacy gave parent-child relations an altogether different cast than is common in modern societies.

Long life, as well as other important social changes, has had a decided effect on adolescence and youth. Not only has adolescence become institutionalized through the mechanism of compulsory education, but youth has been accorded a status out of proportion to its social attributes or its material contribution to society. Lifting the shadow of death and virtually assuring long life has given youth a view of life that is conducive to the exercise of freedom to plan, prepare, and experiment with life in a way never thought possible.

Not only has youth gained a new freedom from the elimination of death due to infectious disease, but they also have freedom from a quick transition into adulthood. The postponement of death along the life course allows for increased leisure, sometimes forced affluence, a greater degree of expansiveness in outlook, and the possibility of envisioning plans for the future.

It seems an anomaly of recent history that at a time when the average youth had the longest future life possible, a significant portion of youth in the 1960s rejected all thought of or plans for the future. They demanded that life be lived in the here and now; pleasure was to be the order of the day, and seemingly the only end worthy of effort. "Do your own thing" was a popular slogan.

A sizeable minority of youth during the late 1960s or early 1970s protested against the exploration of the past. The study of history was deemed a waste of time. To be hung up on the past was denounced as irrelevant. Correspondingly, the tacit acceptance of violence and terror as effective tools of social change show an incredible ignorance of the consequences of violence revealed by human history. Moreover, if ever there was a time when the old adage "eat, drink, and be merry for tomorrow we may die" is not applicable, it is now!

A child's first view of the world is provided by adults, and under high mortality schedules, adults can be little else but cynical regarding the future of anyone's life, not least their own. Adult cynicism has undoubtedly been an important feature of socialization in past times. The reference in Chapter 3 to childhood learning regarding the imminence of death, illustrated by the A.B.C.s, gives testimony to the pervasiveness of this aspect of socialization. An approach to life that rests on the precarious and early end of life is no longer necessary or functional. The partial change in such cynicism is revealed in the sincerity of parental planning and heavy psychological and material investments made in children. This has contributed to the openness and optimism characteristic of contemporary American youth.

Although the present almost idyllic experience of childhood among the middle class may have a few negative consequences, it is a vast improvement over a life that constantly experienced death and its pervasive consequences. In the late 1960s, one social commentator stated that the current youthful rebellion resulted from the clash between the "unbelievable happiness of childhood" and the more demanding features of the adult world.[2] The improvement and lengthening of childhood and the subsequent stage of adolescence through which one can pass without many real reminders of one's own mortality gives the early years of modern men and women the basis for an expanded view of life, as well as an orientation toward the future.

Although the social consciousness of youth has long been characterized by a self-conception of immortality, the actual decline in the experience of death and the slow and almost imperceptible loss of one's age peers have strengthened this conception. The relatively high rates for accidental death for American youth seventeen and eighteen years of age is an exception.

The age-old realities of life still impinge on youth, although some have changed their form. Attempts on the part of parents to enlighten their children to the sober realities of life have diminished. There is little necessity for teaching the young about death. The reality of death is now learned from the omnipresent mass media.

They relate to issues of crime, genocide, and war, but on a level that is mostly abstract and remote. The result is that the search for a meaning to life is taking place earlier than in the past. Ironically, a sign of this is seen in the teenage suicide rate, at a time when premature death by disease is almost nil.

The search for meaning of life is augmented by increases in the intellectual tools of abstract thought, knowledge of the wide variety of human cultures, and the possibilities for new life-styles inherent in greater leisure time. The intensity in the criticisms of traditions and older modes of life by contemporary youth (and young adults) is consistent with the new dimensions of time and testing of alternatives that longevity and modern society afford.

Long life and the change of perspective on conduct and meaning of youth as a distinct period has not only resulted in the problem of adolescence, but has allowed for a long and pervasive period of education and experimentation with varied occupations and life-styles. This has been done without suffering the penalties imposed on the dabblers or slow bloomers of a former time when middle age began at thirty-five and old age at fifty-five.

The decrease in awareness of death for oneself and one's peers has led to a potential rise in the level of intimacy among youth and young adults, both unmarried and married. Increased closeness of modern relationships has also had its risks. Expectations and intense desires for heightened intimacy and togetherness are sometimes difficult to maintain over an extended time period. Many intimate relationships are disrupted following separation or divorce and result in despair and personal disorganization. The increase in length of life all along the life course has provided the time for long and intimate relationships, but the means for preventing their breakup are often lacking. Long life has increased the possibilities and the risks of heightened intimacy.

The level of intimacy between parents and children has also been greatly affected by the decline in infant and maternal mortality. Childbearing is no longer the great risk that it was in the past. The decline and elimination of many childhood diseases has allowed parents to emotionally invest a great deal of themselves in their children.

Long life thus adds to the potential of increased intimacy of family relationships in childhood, but long life also means that parents and grandparents live much longer. This not only insures a degree of continuity to the intimacy originating in childhood, but adds new risks or hurdles to be overcome. Long life increases the risk of divorce and separation. It also enhances the possibilities for parental interference in the late youth and early adult life of children. Parents are sometimes tempted to recoup their own failures or missed opportunities by attempting to push their children into living out their own desires. In effect, parents may see the possibility of vicariously experiencing the successes of a son or daughter. This may help to make late middle and old age more pleasant, since the longer one lives the more one's successes become apparent. The converse may also occur. It becomes problematic when the parents live long enough to realize that not only have their own lives fallen short of the mark they had dreamed of earlier but their children do not meet the expectations they had hoped for them. For example, a study of mothers (average age sixty-nine) who had experienced the divorce of one or more of their children showed that most of the mothers suffered traumatic, sad, and painful feelings for their children.[3]

Parental concern and domination may help to account for the heavy demands for high level performance, educational and otherwise, placed on children and youth. This applies primarily to those future orientated, goal-striving individuals who comprise an important part of modern industrial society. Parental pressure, domination through unwanted advice, and financial dependence and manipulation are a relatively new pitfall facing youth and young adults. This was much less conceivable when the parents became old in their late fifty's and died within a decade. A new category of elderly, the "young old," and the potential for postponing old age until seventy or seventy-five, will probably increase considerably the power and status of the parental generation. This will make the problem of youthful independence even more of an issue than it is now.

During the eighteenth and nineteenth centuries, age differentiation and special categories of youth and young adulthood were less clearly defined. "Under conditions in which the life course was compressed into a shorter and more homogeneous span, the major transition into adulthood, such as leaving school, entering the labor force, leaving home, marrying, and having children were not so clearly structured as they are today. Except for marriage and the formation of households, they did not even necessarily represent moves toward independent adulthood. The order in which they occurred varied significantly, rather than following a customary sequence."[4]

Active parenthood has a beginning and an ending. The most obvious limits are biological, but there are social limits as well. Bearing and raising children must take place relatively early in the life course. Ordinarily we have only one chance to fulfill parental roles from childbirth to the launching of our children into the adult world. Generally we cannot start a family, stop, and start over again without serious disorganization and disruption.

In terms of the family, long life means beginning and completing the childbearing and rearing phases of life. That is, living through and beyond Hill's six stages of family life: new parents, preschool family, school-age family, family with adolescent, family with young adult, and family as a launching center.[5] Though life has been extended, we have, generally speaking, one opportunity to raise a family from the *new parent* stage through the *launching* stage. This fact has an enormous effect on our identity in terms of adequacy, success, or failure in a set of demanding and and socially important roles. It is a once in a lifetime experience and cannot be redone. With long life, one is forced to live with the results of one's choices and endeavors. Parents are principal actors in most families and view themselves as such, though modern social conditions have diminished and even eliminated many of their traditional functions. The importance of the parental role and the nonrepetitive nature of the role make it reasonable to believe that the change to the postparental life may initially be viewed as the loss of an important role. Therefore, the distinctive role changes involved in the aging process preclude opting for family and parenthood a second time.

Extended life means that a large proportion of each generation live through the child-rearing phases, and live long enough to see the results of earlier efforts and actions. This may involve feelings of elation and pride or senses of failure and guilt. In most cases, parents will find that their children do not grow up exactly as they had planned. Most dreams are not fulfilled, though frequently the results may be equal or superior to the early dreams. Having the privilege of living long enough to view the results of one's family life and career require a different set of personality characteristics from that needed for a short or precarious life when long life is viewed as a lucky accident.

Long life substantially changes the nature of "the moving perspective in which the person sees his life as a whole and interprets the meaning of his various attitudes, actions and the things which happen to him."[6] The change in perspective occurs as individuals live a long life and because a great part of each birth cohort lives on as part of a generation. We are used to hearing about the possibilities for political influence and power that lie in the increased number of elderly. However, it is not only the gain in an elderly population that is important, but rather, the diminished losses through death of youth, middle, and late middle-aged cohorts that gives long life its importance. Maintaining the size of age cohorts over a long part of the life course increases their social impact. The increased number of age peers changes the social composition of society. As such, we can hypothesize that the nature of conventional perspectives that are held in relation to child rearing, family roles, and aging will be subtantially altered. We are in a transition period.

The fact that the family roles and identities comprise such an important part of peoples lives, make abrupt change difficult if not impossible. Family roles differ from other major roles and identities, such as those in the occupational areas. According to middle class perspective, the work career is viewed as a single period. It begins at approximately age twenty-three to twenty-eight years, after a lengthy formal education, and continues for about thirty-five to forty years.

Long Life, Middle Age, and the Later Years

One of the major consequences of long life for the middle-aged is the redefinition of the beginning of old age. The change in definition has extended the beginning of old age, thereby lengthening the middle age. The new gerontological concept of "young old" illustrates this change. While this has expanded the possibilites for a new life in the midst of the life course, it has also brought social and psychological problems. Since middle age is the period immediately prior to old age, it is subject to some of the problems that anticipation of old age may bring.

Social gerontologists have devoted some efforts toward the social psychological and personality characteristics of the middle-aged. Neugarten wrote, "We are impressed . . . with reflection as a striking characteristic of the mental life of middle-aged persons: the stock-taking, the heightened introspection, and above all, the structuring and restructuring of experience — that is, the conscious processing of new information in the light of what one has already learned; and turning one's proficiency to the achievement of desired ends."[7] That such a finding is unique to twentieth century modern men and women may be debatable. However, the increased number of older people, the decreased depletion of their age peers (cohorts), and the influence on life perspective resulting from the change in the timing of death has altered the quality of middle-age life.

Longevity makes the characteristics of middle and old age of particular significance for man's future. For example, at what point in the life course does "reflection as a striking characteristic of the mental life of middle-aged person" occur? If it is a positive characteristic, and Neugarten implies this, it should be determined how and when it comes about. Long life occurs in societies that demand social participation in numerous roles at the same time, and these frequently change greatly in the course of long life. In meeting the discontinuity of rapid social change, it might be beneficial to develop or induce reflection before the onset of middle age. It is obvious that this middle age characteristic can be observed in some individuals who are far from biological middle age. One of the consequences of long life is the need to continuously adjust one's self-concept to social reality. Reflection might facilitate this kind of adjustment, and aid in resolving other problems of middle age.

Both Butler and Neugarten refer to an "inner sense of the life cycle" that is apparently reached as men and women become middle-aged. Butler describes this sense of time as — "neither the same as the average expectable life cycle nor the same as a personal sense of identity, although it is related to both. It is a subjective feel for the life cycle as a whole, its rhythm, its variability, and the relation of this to the individual's sense of himself. This inner sense seems to be a necessary personal achievement in order for the individual to orient himself wherever he happens to be on the life cycle."[8]

This conception is related to the awareness of the fact that around the midpoint of our expected length of life, we begin to accept our own mortality. This occurs, generally speaking, between the years of thirty-five and forty, about half way through our expected length of life. This awareness contributes to our concern about the timing of major events and accomplishments, either those in the past or those projected into the future. It gives a new aspect to our sense of self, a sense of our position within our personal or family history.

Our sense of the life course varies by culture and historical time. When and how it develops is the result of the interplay of individual lives and the social structure as expressed in the age norms that help regulate the individual's passage through the life course. Neugarten has stated that "the age norm system not only provides mechanisms for allocating new recruits to the major social roles, it also creates an ordered predictable life course; it creates time tables and it sets boundaries for acceptable behaviors in successive life stages."[9] That is, "adults carry around in their heads, whether or not they can verbalize it, a set of anticipations of the normal expectable life cycle. . . . They make plans and set goals along a time-line shaped by these expectations."[10] This provides an important part of the social structure governing social life, and contributes the framework for each person's inner sense of the life cycle. This structure is vitally effected by demographic phenomena, such as death rates. A general awareness of the choronology of death and the normal lifespan impinge on the social structure as well as on our individual consciousness. The frequency of death and whether or not it is viewed as imminent leads to a shorter life perspective. It also introduces a seemingly random disruption in parts of the social structure as in the family, close and distant, as well as the assassination of public figures.

Individuals frequently interpret these critical events as having special import for their own lives. For example, a woman whose mother died at an early age may have fears that she may also die leaving her own child without a mother. For some, such a tragic death may inhibit child bearing altogether. The event of death and when it occurs in the life course seriously effects the social norms of society, as well as individuals and families. It may alter our view of the way we anticipate certain sequences of events.

In transition to the new age of longevity, there is impressionistic evidence that middle age frequently signals the onset of a relatively long and depressing period of continuous physical decline. The cult of youth with its symbols of physical beauty, athletic prowess, sexual capacity, and physical endurance stimulates a negative view of middle age. Emphasis on the primacy of youth has roots in our history. Literary sources from Colonial America reveal a deep "association between age and physical depletion in the minds of the New Englanders, 'infirmity,' 'deformity,' 'weakness,' 'natural decay,' 'ill savors,' 'the scent of rottenness,' — such terms recur throughout their writings on old age."[11] Concern with physiological aging made sense in a society that relied so heavily on physical exertion. Strong arms and nimble legs were very important in those times.

Not unlike his predecessors, the contemporary middle-aged person frequently experiences ambivalence, apprehension, and despair as the biological evidence of aging becomes fully apparent and can no longer be hidden or ignored. This may apply primarily to those who are active athletically and who possess a strong identity with the physical aspect of youth, a substantial group in the American population. This is discussed further in the section on "Long Life and the Problem of Losses." Demos has commented,* "Nowadays physical aging is typically, and often powerfully, associated with the passage from youth to middle age; here, indeed, lies an important part of what we call the 'midlife crisis.' "[12] In the early years of the country, the same crisis signalled the beginning of old age. That such should be the case is not surprising since work and family responsibilities are usually great, and evidence of rising success in the middle classes is most apparent in the middle age period. Middle age roles require intense activity. The period may be characterized as the time to "work hard and play hard." During this period, most people become aware of the fact that this is also the time for reaching one's peak, which unfortunately reinforces the conception that life represents a trajectory, rising to midlife and then declining thereafter. This is a view that has done much to curtail and even destroy the later years.

Although middle age life is viewed as the peak or prime of life, it may not be particularly joyous or even satisfactory. It is the period when references to being in a rat race abound. On the average, it is the period of relatively low marital satisfaction. Marriages that have reached fifteen or twenty years show a rise in divorce rates.[13] Early heart attacks, midlife diabetic episodes, and social and psychological problems involving young adult children develop. In a recent study emphasizing the positive possibilities in old age, the author writes, "Middle age, perhaps the worst of times, is often the time of greatest stress and anxiety. It is then that there is the rising sense of frustra-

---

From a Little Commonwealth: Family Life in Plymouth Colony by John Demos. Copyright© 1970 by Oxford University Press, Inc. Reprinted by permission.

tion, fear, and defeat, the awareness that fame and fortune will never come, that the best of life is past. Middle-aged people have fearsome double burdens — paying for the support of both younger and older generations, juggling the values of one against the other, feeling ambivalent or guilty toward both — all the while that the prospect of their own old age stares them in the face."[14] Although the period may often lack great joy and satisfaction, it is the period in which the quintessential determinants of success or failure for the rest of the life course take place. According to conventional wisdom, childhood and youth are preparatory, and late middle and old age represent "inevitable decline."

Longevity helps to provide the potential for long marriages, but also increases the possibility of separation and divorce. Whether or not marriages stay intact or end in divorce, the necessity of making family related role changes, and adapting to new situations remains a part of life, though somewhat different in detail. A marriage that endures moves into the post parental period. The decline of the parent role and the establishment of life as a couple again are important and, in many cases, positive. This part of the life course can provide individuals with new possibilities. Work may even be intensified since responsibility for day-to-day care of children is gone. Wives may have time and energy for new or intensified work careers. Hobbies and special recreational plans may be pursued, and new ventures in work, business, travel, or volunteer activities may be initiated. Early retirement and plans for a second career may occur at this time.

At the interpersonal level, some of the changes that take place may result in the fading of old friendships and associations, especially those that have been based on interests and concerns relating to children and family. In the early and middle years of adulthood, children, neighborhood affairs, schools, holidays, and family vacations provide an important area of mutual concern. Many adults friendships form over these concerns. However, when the children are gone, and the resident family reverts to only husband and wife, many of the former interests may diminish or cease to exist. Thus, the traditional notion that "old friends are the best friends" may not apply. Other old friends are lost to death, incapacity, or change of residence. Nevertheless, some of the insecurities resulting from social losses due to aging, as well as the notion that old friends are best, may inhibit couples from seeking new ones. Middle to late middle age is the beginning of a period of life that may last at least ten to fifteen years. The potential need for developing new friends and associations poses a personal challenge that many middle-aged people are not well prepared to meet. By middle age, most people have a fully established family and kin group, friendship circle, and work group. When circumstances are satisfactory, few venture much beyond the boundaries of their established groups. Therefore, the attitudes and skills needed in developing new relationships are left dormant. The prevalent conception, however, that the life course forms a trajectory and that the last half of life is all "down hill," inhibits planning and cultivating new friends. Long life has increased the importance of the attitudes and interpersonal skills that make these kinds of changes possible. Other challenges to personal capabilities and commitments face the middle-aged.

Middle-aged children may find themselves in the position of having to becomes aides and resources to their aging parents. The ability to become a resource to parents, without creating a pattern of role reversal, is referred to as *filial maturity*.[15] Hess and Markson state that "A new set of tasks confronts the middle-aged offspring of aged parents: to act as guides and protectors in dealing with the bureaucracy that now surrounds family life and aging. The children can intervene on behalf of parents, ensure their entitlements, and deal with red tape."[16] To achieve a positive level of filial maturity is frequently a difficult task, and poses social psychological problems that defy solution. Other problems relating to role conflict emerge in this period.

For example, in the family wherein the wife and mother has invested the bulk of her emotional energies in children and family affairs, but has also worked in a job outside the family, the wife-mother-worker roles can create conflict. The wife-mother-worker roles may, in fact, create more role conflict than husband-father-worker roles. Although the husband's work role often takes more "role space" and is more dominating than most of the woman's roles, it generally involves less conflict in the family. For many women the discontinuities and conflict in the wife-mother-worker roles ultimately result in a better adjustment to old age. Role discontinuity and change during middle age enhance coping abilities.

A recent twelve-year study found that the loss of a spouse adversely affected husbands much more than wives.[17] Men whose spouses died were much more likely to die during the following few years than men who were still married. In turn, men who remarried improved their chances of living longer. The death of a spouse had little or no effect on the mortality of women. For reasons that are not well understood, women are more able to adapt to the loss of their spouse. The data further showed that the effect of a wife's death appeared to reflect "A chronic, long-term problem of being alone, rather than an immediate response to the death itself."[18]

Aging, Embarrassment, and Failure

Considerable research and theorizing has been done in dealing with the question of the decline in social participation of the aged. In some instances, a decline in social participation may be more closely associated with fears relating to embarrassment and personal failure rather than apathy, lack of interest, or physical energy.

When queried, however, the elderly often give excuses such as health, expense, or difficulties with transportation. The problem of embarrassment rests on the maintenance of an identity and its corresponding role. This is particularly important to the aged since crucial role changes occur as aging takes place, such as nonvoluntary retirement from the work role and widowhood. Relying on the work of Gross and Stone, Miller writes the following:

> If a rationale for the activity by the aged is to be maintained and an identity developed, the person, once he participates in some activity, must be capable of supporting a role in the group throughout the social interactions and performances required of a participant. Identity, writes Gross and Stone, 'must be continually reaffirmed, must be maintained, and provision made for repair in case of breakdown' (Gross and Stone, unpublished). The result of identity breakdown — a social occurrence which belies what the person has announced he is, and what he is capable of, by assuming the role of participant — is embarrassment. In turn, embarrassment makes continued role performance difficult and undermines the foundation of the new identity.[19]

Embarrassment can occur as the result of a *faux pas*, which reveals to others that the person is dated in knowledge and behavior.[20] A person may be unable to respond appropriately due to economic, family, or health problems. This is particularly apparent when seen in relation to physical incapacity due to aging. Losses in hearing, sight, and steadiness of hand, etc. may keep the aged person from going out to dinner at a friend's house or to a restaurant. Spilling the coffee, dribbling gravy on one's tie or blouse, inability to read the menu or bill, or hear enough to converse with others may be too embarrassing to bear. Thus, the possibility of embarrassment limits social participation and elderly individuals may exclude themselves from social interaction with others, sometimes even from their immediate family, peers, or members of their own age cohort.[21]

When embarrassment occurs, it inhibits the individual from the continued performance of the role in question. This is due to the presumption of a spoiled identity and the undermining of the assumptions that the participants make about each other in a role performance. The aged, however, like crippled people, are often considered the most likely to fail and are destined to suffer embarrassment. Sometimes attempts are made to arrange the social situation so that the chance of failure and embarrassment is decreased. "The problem of embarrassment and its ramifications are avoided by providing the aging participant with a social role within the system which he can maintain. . . ."[22] The social definition of the roles and situations to be controlled, in order to avoid embarrassment, place limits on the aged, by self-limitation as well as the limits imposed by well meaning others. With the long history of negative connotations associated with age and the contemporary cult of activity-oriented rejuvenescence a situation has developed in which the assumed limitations and foibles of age may be overestimated on the part of those who are young, as well as the old. Unfortunately, the aged often view themselves negatively in much the same way as do the young. This results in the acceptance by the elderly of a somewhat circumscribed set of relatively unimportant, uninteresting, failure-proof roles, such as helper, aides, spectator, residents, hobbyists, and so on. Narrow limitations on role performance is one of the consequences of the negative definition of aging, which also contributes to the maintenance of such definitions. In general, younger persons often underestimate the capabilities of the elderly, which leads to frustration and distress for both old and young.

Loneliness, Friendship, and Intimacy

Studies report that loneliness and boredom are also social psychological phenomena associated with aging. On an extended scale, loneliness may result from long life as much as it does from the individuality and pluralism of modern industrial society. In contrast to the times when life was precarious, short, and demanding in the single-minded pursuit of subsistence and survival, there is now time for reflexive thought that can result in loneliness. One can argue that long life calls for greater inner resources in meeting the added loneliness, perhaps with the aim of at least changing it to a more emotionally neutral aloneness. Increased loneliness may be one of the consequences of affluence and longevity.

As with loneliness, extra time in old age may lead to boredom. This is frequently true of the working classes, as well as others who have been unable to develop interests that could be cultivated upon retirement.[23] Boredom indicates an inability to move from the work role to the retirement role. These earlier trends appear to be changing with a growing elderly population that is more educated and affluent. Curiously, one study of older people revealed that of the nearly 40 percent who expressed a desire for new activities, "fully three-fourths did not know why they did not undertake new activities."[24] There is some impressionistic evidence that aging lowers the intensity of human relationships, as well as other emotional aspects of life. Such a change, if left uncompensated for, may help to account for the apparent apathy found among some of the elderly.

Friendship and intimacy are important components in the maintenance of a positive self-identity and assist in meeting some of the losses that occur for the aged. In a study of older people, those who belonged to a close knit friendship group considered themselves old much less often than those who did not belong.[25] To consider oneself old in present-day industrial society seems to connote a kind of social psychological decline or defeat. To avoid such an identity implies a positive adjustment to the problems and limitations of old age.

Friendship group membership not only tends to slow a self-identification with being old, but offers continuity and stability in a world of discontinuity. Blau states that "stability of the network of relationship within a group of friends or co-workers prevents mutual awareness of gradual alterations that take place in each of the participants, particularly if these changes in the person do not interfere with his ability to share in the activities of the group. Consequently, the recurrent gatherings of the same people lend a sense of continuity in the life of each participant."[26]

Another study dealt with intimacy and morale in old age.[27] An intimate relationship, such as having a confidant, was found to have a significant effect on the morale of the aged. An intimate relationship proved to be more than having a great amount of interaction with others. Even such losses as becoming widowed were significantly buffered by having a confidant. The prolongation of life into old age has increased the potentiality for gaining and retaining a friendship group or confidant. The slowing of the depletion of old age peer groups (and birth cohorts) gives existent ones the possibility of remaining reasonably intact for a longer time than in the past. In earlier times, those who grew old were often left without age peers for the last ten to fifteen years of their lives. Thus, the kinds of social support that Blau refers to is of relatively recent origin, at least for the mass of the aging population.

Presuming that major cardiac diseases and cancer will be conquered and no diseases take their place, each age cohort will remain intact longer. However, as each cohort reaches very old age, it will proceed to die off more quickly than presently. If and when this occurs, the demise of a given cohort of aged will take place at such a rate that a new set of social and psychological problems for the very old will develop. Though longevity has altered the timing and consequences of death, its problematic and crisis characteristics will probably continue in the foreseeable future. The prolongation of life, however, has provided the basis for vast improvements in the later years.

Long Life, the Self, Competence, and Control

Long life provides the conditions required for the perspective needed to fully develop and realize a sense of self, both socially and physiologically. For the individual, long life can contribute to an increased freedom from some of the constraints of society and culture. One who has lived through the major phases of life, such as family, work, education, retirement, or is still working in the later years, has in a sense "had it all," although such a view is only valid in a society that views life as a trajectory and defines the end as a decline prior to death. Nevertheless, as the definition of old age has become more vague and indeterminant, many defy the traditional assumptions about old age and exercise a level of personal freedom that gives them a new and expanded sense of self. This can also result in a new life-style for the end of the life course.

When we have lived for a long time, we may come to see society as less compelling, less a part of ourselves. This can generate the freedom to deal more adequately with society in objective terms. The individual can then make choices, more self-consciously, based on personal considerations. He or she can be less coerced by convention and fear of social reprisal. Many of the potential reprisals appear less compelling when one has had the experience of a marriage career, parental career, and work career. This may not apply to the lowest socioeconomic classes, but seems to appear in the middle and upper classes.

The increased psychological freedom and feeling of ability to direct one's own life is creating conditions for social change that are not always in the direction pushed by social conventions, but by one's own self identity and desire. As individuals exercise freedom of choice in old age, portions of the population will collectively learn to view society as being more tolerant, and an awareness that conventions are not equally constraining at all points along the life course will emerge. The vagueness of the old age role has left a social vacuum. Increasing numbers of vigorous, concerned, and "ageless" people are beginning to use the freedom allowed by the lack of a specific role. The vagueness of an elderly role may not be as detrimental as some social gerontologists have argued, especially in a period of transition from a relatively short precarious life to a more stable longer life. When more elderly begin to exercise the available freedom of choice, greater heterogeneity and diversity of behavior will occur. A heterogeneous social world provides the basis for tolerance, freedom, and social change. These are important prerequisites for improving the end of the life course.

We have recently been through a period when the young made strong demands for the freedom to choose. Over the next two decades, we will be in transition from modestly educated cohorts of aged to an increased number of healthier, better educated, involved "young old" people moving into the ranks of the retired, part-time employed, or new careerists. Their large numbers will have a substantial effect in realizing the demands for greater freedom of choice. The search of the elderly for optional life-styles involving work, leisure, and family responsibility may be different from that of youth, but the exercise of choice is the crucial element. This new and more experienced older segment of the population will add to the collective effects of the young in the formation of new folkways, laws, policies, and norms in dealing with the expanding dimensions of life presented by longevity in a modern technological society. Neugarten wrote, "The young-old are likely to want greater options for what generally might be called an 'age irrelevant' society, one in which arbitrary constraints based on chronological age are removed, and in which all individuals have opportunities consonant with their needs, desires, and abilities, whether they be young or old. Overall, as the young-old articulate their needs and desires, the emphasis is likely to be upon improving the generality of life and upon increasing the choice of life-style."[28]

The ability to make the personal choices that create freedom of action for the elderly is dependent on flexibility and adaptability of those who become old. Our current rhetoric of crisis at various stages of life, including the so-called midlife crisis, has connotations regarding the incapacity of the individual to change.[29] As is known, aging does not cause an incapacity to change, but if the individual "is unable to cognitively or emotionally perceive, accept, or use new ideas, techniques, life-styles, and values, we observe a . . . stereotypical reproduction of earlier attempts toward solution of occupational or private problems, and are fatigued by the redundancy and connected evasion of inadequate problem solution."[30] Long life provides such a lengthy period of old age that the rejection of the stereotypic view of aging becomes both socially necessary, as well as possible. As Parsons reminds us, the fifteen or more years that we can expect to live after age sixty-five is not a "trivial matter either for the individual or the society."[31]

One of the implications of this analysis is that continuity and permanence in the form of a rigid set of sequences involving education, marriage, family, work career, and retirement will frequently fail to meet the needs of long life. This poses a rather serious paradox. There is little doubt that current stereotypic conceptions of the life course require that the flexibility of youth be diminished enough to allow long-term commitments in adulthood. Labouvie-Vief states, ". . . the hallmark of adulthood is commitment and responsibility. Careers must be started, intimacy bonds formed, children raised. In short, in a world of a multitude of logical possibilities, *one* course of action must be adopted. This conscious commitment to one pathway and the deliberate disregard of other logical choices may mark the onset of adult cognitive maturity."[32] Nevertheless, a study of the socialization process of women and how it affected successful aging, concluded that "If the theory that impermanence and discontinuity over the adult life cycle exerts a direct effect upon positive adjustment to old age is valid, then a new system of career flexibility should be adopted as the new battle cry by men and women."[33] In effect, the flexibility and adaptability needed for a successful long life in a rapidly changing society must be learned through experience all along the life course. This conclusion conforms to our current conceptions of the lifelong process of socialization.

Precisely what portions of midlife must be devoted to permanence and continuity and flexibility and adaptability is presently undeterminable. Agreement might be gained on the notion that twenty or so years in young adulthood and midlife, which is devoted to childbearing and rearing as well as the initial work career, requires the greatest measure of permanence and continuity. In turn, a substantial part of youth and late middle and old age would require the least. The self-esteem and confidence needed to shift between continuity and change is different from that required by a life of permanence and stability. Irrespective of the development of the kind of self that will evolve due to long life, the maintenance of a strong and stable self-concept is an important ingredient in successful aging.

After a long life in which one has gained a substantial level of competence and exercised considerable control over life one's self-image becomes closely related to a self-perception of competence and control. The earlier reference to losses that lead to embarrassment and loneliness underscore this point. If one lives in a society that seems to strip one of control and systematically denies one's competence, the maintenance of self-esteem becomes difficult at best.

Various losses associated with aging, both social psychological and physiological, easily result in loss of control and independence. This diminishes self-image. Although one's self-concept is in continuous development and changes in meeting the circumstances of life a certain core of personality tends to remain stable. A crucial element of this core is the feeling of competence and control gained by functioning acceptably in the social roles that are expected and viewed as desirable. Middle age is recognized as the important period when the sense of one's capabilities, control, and independence are most fully developed. This is true for both occupation and family life. When a sense of competence and control develop, the changes associated with old age can be met, and long life can be more satisfactory instead of grim.

An analysis by Arnold Rose of the social function of voluntary associations may have relevance for the development of some of the coping abilities needed to maintain a self-image that can meet the exigencies of long life.[34] He argued that participation in voluntary associations served to give people a feeling that they mattered and that they could exercise some control over their lives. Individuals who were submerged in bureaucratic work settings could gain a feeling of having influence and could even assume leadership positions through voluntary association memberships. This may partially account for the growth in personal adjustment and in the structuring of their social life that appears when the participating elderly are compared to those who do not.[35] Such involvement ranges from religious organizations to hobby and leisure groups. Rose argued that any kind of voluntary association membership could serve those whose work is closely structured. The development of a self that can maintain the independence and control needed for a satisfactory long life is made increasingly difficult in a society that trivializes and neglects the elderly.

The problems relating to the maintenance of competence and control, on the scale of the larger society, were of less salience in the past than in the present. In preindustrial times, most of the elderly worked and maintained control over the family's economic assets until they died. Relatively few reached our current new categories of *old-old* (75-85) or the *extremely elderly* (over 85). The problems of adjustment and life satisfaction in old age appear to have been less when death decimated each cohort at all ages of the life course and left relatively few to become old. This, however, was not true for the poor and destitute. Thus, long life has intensified the problem, but may also have made the solution possible. The solution to providing the elderly with a good and fruitful life to the end of their days may turn out to be just as difficult as it was to extend life itself in the sense that it took decades rather than months or years.

How does long life affect the maintenance of a sense of control over one's own life? Essentially, one's cohort members remain living, thus giving one a peer group in old age. The existence of intact peer groups well into old age has the potential for helping maintain a stable and satisfactory self-concept. This has increased the prospect of maintaining a sense of control. The sharing of the biological consequences of age and gaining coping information through peer behavior and interest give one the breadth of perspective, techniques, and ideas needed for coping with the losses of aging. Research findings show that the elderly who feel in control of their lives are those who are more capable of meeting the stresses of aging.[36]

Long Life and the Problem of Losses

Against a strong belief in the preeminence of youth, aging poses many new personal problems regarding losses of one kind or another. Many of these problems require new attitudes and new coping approaches. Some of them may involve major changes in earlier life-styles, attitudes, and values relating to a successful life. Much of the behavior and activity that may be productive in a short life may be detrimental in a long life.

Our store of social knowledge regarding the best approach and type of behavior needed to insure a long good life to the end is not well known, or at least not well articulated. The problems of the aged have, however, been energetically studied and described. Some of the problems commonly discussed are not particularly related to the effects of long life, nor the direct results. The present discussion will be limited to those problems that are especially affected by the increase in length of life for large numbers of people.

Traditionally, long life has been viewed as an experience in which losses seem to far outweigh gains. The declines in the physiological functioning of the body are portrayed by the graphs that are found in books and pamphlets dealing with gerontology that reveal the descending curves characterizing metabolic rates, liver functions, physical strength, lung capacity, etc. Similar charts are found for various mental capacities such as memory. However, recent consideration of this display of age decrements are beginning to indicate that much of this measurable decline has relatively little to do with what is biologically necessary to pursue a satisfactory life.

Many of these losses are little needed in functioning adequately until very late in life unless one is strongly oriented toward a definition of self in biological terms with an emphasis on youthful physical performance.

Despite the controversy of whether it is age or disease that imposes the major physical decrements on the elderly, the fact remains that serious losses occur as a result of various disabilities. This is particularly true in connection with the senses, such as hearing, sight, and physical mobility. One student of old age poses the problem in terms of the orientation people have toward their own bodies. Whether an individual approaches the fact of physical deterioration from the point of view of *body preoccupation* or *body transcendence* will have much to do with his response to old age. "For people to whom pleasure and comfort mean predominantly physical well-being, this (declining health) may be the gravest, most mortal of insults. There are many such people whose older years seem to move in a decreasing spiral, centered around their growing preoccupation with the state of their bodies. There are other people, however, who suffer just as painful physical unease, yet who enjoy life greatly. . . . In their value system, social and mental sources of pleasure and self respect may transcend physical comfort, alone."[37] Peck contends that the choice of how one views one's own physical decline is an important aspect of old age. It seems apparent that the social and psychological factors dictating such a choice emerge and develop throughout middle age or earlier.

Since long life not only allows but necessitates a confrontation with physical decline and susceptibility to disease, the development of attitudes towards one's physical self becomes an important facet of everyone's life. It is a facet that many men and women in the past did not live long enough to experience, at least not in relation to advanced age. The emergence of new attitudes and values relative to physical decline may have considerable impact on other aspects of life. One such aspect is the adulation of youth — a salient orientation of many Americans and Europeans. Modification in valuing youthful physical characteristics might allow for an increased value being placed upon mental and social characteristics. Since these characteristics decline least with advancing age, such a shift would be functional for the long life that most men and women will experience.

In contrast to the usual assumptions about physical decline and incapacity that form the stereotype of the aged, there is evidence that greater efforts toward the maintenance of the human body may forestall the stereotype of the elderly as being weak and infirm.

On the basis of a one-year program of exercise for a group of men seventy years and over, de Vries reports a great improvement in general fitness and health. The bodily reactions of these men resembled those of men in their forties.[38] "Such evidence suggests that much of the decline in abilities that does occur among the aged may be due more to declining exercise and activity than to any inevitable aging process itself."[39] In addition to the possibility that a new and more comprehensive approach to exercise in middle and old age may improve life, a concern with diet is also beginning to have an impact on everyday habits and behavior.

Exercise, diet, and possibly other maintenance kinds of behavior will probably increase in importance with an awareness of the potentiality and consequences of longevity. Control of disease is often closely tied to these aspects of physical life, though in some cases are quite independent of exercise and diet. The rise in preventative medicine and concern with "community health" are evidence of the more comprehensive nature of advanced medical thinking.

It is quite possible that a number of the disabilities and assumed characteristics of old age are diseases that may be controllable in the future. Though cancer and heart disease are currently the greatest killers, the prospect that arteriosclerosis may be prevented or reversed could mean that life for many of the elderly would significantly change. Effective prevention or control of maladies such as arthritis and rheumatism would have an added impact. Butler states that ". . . . we have found evidence to suggest that many manifestations heretofore associated with aging per se, reflect instead medical illness, personality variables, and social-cultural effects."[40] Though the possibility for a radical scientific breakthrough in dealing with the disease-linked characteristics of advanced age currently seems slight, even small advances might have large-scale consequences. Longevity has created great numbers of aged people. The increased heterogenity in style of life and the social and psychological response to old age have already resulted in important changes.

Two hundred years ago, relatively few lived long enough to suffer extreme loss in the functioning of sensory organs. The loss of hearing

and sight have such profound social consequences that their importance cannot be minimized. The decline in vision is the least serious
since the use of glasses and contact lenses can correct for substantial
loss. The same cannot be said for hearing. It is estimated that by age
sixty-five, about 50 percent of the men and 30 percent of the women
in the United States have suffered hearing losses that hinder social
interaction.[41] Furthermore, there is evidence that the elderly who
suffer severe hearing or speech impairment are even more likely to
be placed in old age homes and chronic disease institutions than
those who are incontinent and bedridden.[42] Unfortunately, the
effectiveness of electronic hearing aids is sometimes minimal at best.
The further development of electronic hearing aids and medical procedures that deal with hearing loss could do much to improve life for
the elderly. The rapid increase in the population of those over eighty
should provide adequate justification for increased research support.

The great decline in hearing and sight appears to be connected
with our environment. In certain parts of the Sahara desert where
the usual sounds of modern society are almost entirely absent, "men
and women in their seventies have a hearing ability almost equal to
that of the young — and far superior to the hearing capacity of their
age peers in the urban industrial West."[43] It is also possible
genetically, that a considerable number of humans are poorly
designed to live seven, eight, or nine decades. It has always been
assumed that aging inevitably deprives one of sensory acuity,
though relatively little has been done to deal with the problem, or
develop new techniques to correct these insufficiencies.

Other losses that are more crucial for men than for women are
the changes that occur in ability to perform sexually. For many men
this is an unmistakable sign of aging, one that is frequently viewed
with desperation, and creates intense resistance to the anticipation of
the aging process. Since aging is expected to curtail or end all sexual
activity, relatively little is known about the actual decrements
related to age. Since sexual performance is rarely discussed and is
generally limited as a subject for serious study, little of the available
knowledge is being utilized. The actual physiological losses may be
quite minimal. A longitudinal study is necessary over an extended
period of time. For example, the social and psychological effects of
being born in the cohort of 1890 compared with one born in 1945
could reveal immense differences in the attitudes, values, and expec-

tations involving sex in the later years. Irrespective of the possible lengthening of the period of sexual activity for both males and females, it was found that somewhere in the seventh and eighth decade of life, the vast majority of males are destined to lose their abilites to perform in conventional ways. Physical closeness and intimate caressing seem to offer an important substitute for active sexual performance for the very old. However, there is reason to assume that active sex, like so many other activities traditionally associated with youth, is and will continue to be extended to a later age than in the past.

The losses involving sight, hearing, and sex require considerable adaptation and reorientation during the latter part of the life course. These losses, if progressive and extreme, result in a serious decline in all kinds of stimulation from the external environment. Not only is social interaction affected, but stimulation from nature, mass media, music, art, theatre, and many other areas are curtailed. The result can mean isolation, boredom, and paranoid ideations. Such consequences are much more likely under circumstances of long life than under previous mortality schedules. Long life will continue to add to this population unless medical science and technology begin to find solutions. The same can be said for the limitations on mobility imposed by diseases such as arthritis. A crash program for minimizing such biological losses might significantly change the lives of a large elderly population. Such a program could have a far greater social "payoff" than present-day cancer research endeavors. Currently, the disabled elderly must cope with these prospects under adverse conditions.

Our age-old assumptions about the primacy of youth and the rejection of age have not equipped us to cope with the inevitability of such losses. Our history, in which a relatively short precarious life was the norm, has not yet allowed the development of a perspective and new life course schedules that make adaptation to the biological aspects of aging acceptable.

Another aspect of physical aging, is the necessity of exercising greater control over diet, physical exertion, and sleep. Youth and early adulthood seem to allow the luxury of indulging in excessive amounts of food, drink, and physical strain, and loss of sleep all without apparent consequence. In fact, the feeling that one can indulge and only suffer slight repercussion may be one of the important marks of youth. The neglect of one's biological needs and limitations becomes increasingly costly in terms of health and well-being the older one gets. Even for those who do not view youth as the apex, there are strong social inducements to judge oneself against youthful criteria well into old age. Each age needs to be judged against criteria relating to itself rather than unrealistic youthful and physiologically oriented standards. Some reflection will reveal that there are very few specific positive criteria available for judging performance among the elderly.

This point is of great significance because the physical decrements of aging, however they develop in the near future, may now last for many years. This is not a trivial part of life, but is often wasted by isolation and boredom. If improvements are not forthcoming, it may mean that the elderly will continue to equivocate in their attitudes toward death.

The majority of the aged do not particularly fear death and come to accept its approach with a calm attitude, some even welcoming it. This may be due to the fact that life has become meaningless. If this is the case, as claimed by Beauvoir, long life can be viewed as a mixed blessing.[44] Somewhat indicative of the psychological problems faced by the aged are the levels of drug abuse, alcoholism, and suicide that exist among the elderly. Estimates indicate that 10 to 15 percent have serious alcoholic problems. Drug problems, relating to the use of tranquilizers, have emerged in recent years.[45] The easy use of tranquilizers as a way of dealing with problems of the aged has begun to gain national attention. Heavy usage frequently leads to physical and/or emotional dependence.[46] This response to problems has been encouraged by the inadequate development of reliable knowledge in gerontology and geriatric medicine.

In the United States, the suicides among those over sixty-five years of age account for 17 to 25 percent of the total, whereas the elderly only constitute 11 percent of this population.[47] Suicide rates rise with advancing age among white males, but level off in middle age for females.[48] The personal consequences of poor health, retirement, and widowhood may offer a partial answer to this phenomena. In a sample of elderly suicides in Florida occurring between 1955 and 1963, the largest proportion was from those in the lowest socioeconomic class. Various kinds of social relationships were related to old-age suicide. The involvement of marriage, kin groups, and organizational membership could give life the meaning and interaction that would help to prevent suicides.[49]

During World War II, the suicide rate for men in London declined, allegedly the result of their involvement in useful employment.[50] As such, high suicide rates among the elderly may be related to the social consequences surrounding the later years, at least for white males. Using World Health Organization data, Kruijt found that in countries with a continuously rising age curve, the suicide rate increases with age.[51] Curiously, he also found a "marked decrease" in elderly suicide in Britain, the Commonwealth, and Scandinavia. Two explanations are offered for this trend reversal. First, advances in creating welfare states have improved the living conditions of the elderly. The other is that these decreases occur in countries with high suicide rates for the middle-aged groups. In effect, the low rates for the elderly may be the result of a trough that follows a peak in rates for the preceding age-groups.[52] Thus, it is an artifact of the statistics, which in turn, points to suicide as a problem during the middle years in these advanced, urbanized countries.

Mental disorder is another response to the problems of old age. Estimates indicate that about 10 percent of the aged suffer from disabling mental diseases.[53] The functional disorders, those with no known organic cause, are labelled as either psychoses or neuroses. The most frequent type of cases are related to depressions caused by the physical and social losses incurred in the process of aging. Having difficulties in coping with problems earlier in life add to the likelihood that one will develop a functional disorder in old age.[54] Since many of these disorders are a response to the losses in aging, long life may increase the actual losses, thereby increasing the probability of depression. On the other hand, a long life may help to provide impetus toward making greater attempts to cure the psychological disorders of the elderly, rather than merely assuming that the problems are organic. A frequent medical response is to prescribe tranquilizers. Although there is little increase with age, the proportion of disabling mental illness increases. According to this study, it is the result of an increase in the proportion of organic diseases rather than functional disorders. In effect, long life seems to take a greater toll at the organic level than the sociopsychological level. There is, however, a continous debate regarding the ability of geriatric medicine to distinguish between the treatable and untreatable organic brain disorders. Many diagnoses of organic brain disease are made without physiological evidence of any kind. They are made entirely on the basis of reported behavior and advanced age. Setlin argues that there is no valid and practical test that can clearly differentiate between them.[55] It is clear that a greater societal effort towards research into the causes of the whole range of mental disorders affecting the elderly is long overdue.

It is apparent that present-day psychiatry tends to deal inadequately with the aged. Frequently, the elderly do not get therapy, and if they do, it is often too late. Many feel that consulting a psychiatrist is stigmatizing and stay with their physician (general practitioner or internist) until they can no longer be helped. This is reinforced by the predominant orientation toward the organic nature of old age mental disorder and applies to those who care for the aged as well as the aged themselves. These factors and others have resulted in transforming the psychiatry of aging "into the psychiatry of termination."[56] The older patient tends to be viewed in catastrophic terms; the dominant approach is to reconcile them to loss and the inevitability of pain and depression.[57] Without new approaches and better solutions, more and more elderly will be condemned to losses that curtail and deprive them of control and independence.

The losses in physical endurance and sensory acuity and the appearance of one or more diseases give sharp emphasis to the critical nature of maintaining one's control and independence. One of the most powerful perceptive legacies of young adulthood and middle age is the self-conception of independence and control; as a central component of self-image, it must be maintained in order to meet the stresses of aging.

Psychological stress, some of which begins in middle age, has recently become a subject of concern to gerontologists. Although few research findings are available, important questions are beginning to be asked. Parent writes, ". . . what stress types are encountered by middle age? Is it possible that older adults face loss and chronic sorrow more than they face anxiety provoking threats?"[58] The middle age period frequently involves role losses, such as those involved in the changes of the postparental and the preretirement phases. Losses by death of parents, friends or peers, and children, plus the physiological changes inflicted in the forty-five to sixty-year period, challenge ones former identity. In commenting about these changes and challenges, Parent states, "Coping tasks associated with loss are quite different from those of threat. With irrevokable loss the task is to grieve the loss, accept its finality and restructure one's life without the lost object."[59] In contrast to loss, Parent refers to differences in coping "with threat . . . or challenge to cherished goals, . . ., coping strategies either require (1) direct actions in the form of preparation against harm, attack or avoidance or (2) intrapsychic coping through such methods as attention deployment, defensive reappraisal or wish-fulfillment."[60]

In middle age, it is possible that some stresses become almost chronic and require techniques for coping over the long term. "As the generation most free to inherit society's caretaking duties, the postparental group may prove to face such stresses. In addition, it is possible that situations which were accepted as challenges in younger years might be regarded by their cohort as unchangeable. Coping with chronic problems requires defenses against recurring negative emotions, maintenance of self-esteem, development of models for a new life-style, and the development of access to a reference group whose values and goals support the new life-style."[61] As aging continues, changes in life-style may move in negative as well as positive directions. Role reversal represents a negative approach.

When the perception of loss of control and independence occurs, the phenomena of family role reversal sometimes takes place. Through late middle age, parents give their young adult children more in the way of gifts than they receive. As parents age, this tends to reverse itself and children begin to assume the supportive role held by the parent.[62] This has been called role reversal, a state that is similar to the *sick role*, which is frequently taken by those who become dependent due to illness. In other findings, Lowenthal reports that in tradition-oriented working-class communities, people with prescribed status, like the elderly, receive goods and services from others in the social network according to prescribed rules.[63] It is referred to as a "social economy." Although the reciprocal relationships of Lowenthal's social economy are similar to role reversal, they differ in an important way. Role reversal implies a pathological state of dependence without reciprocity. In contrast, Lowenthal's principle does not imply a pathological state, but rather an appropriate service to those with the status of age. This principle is lacking in some sectors of modern society.

It is apparent that severe loss of income and the physiological problems of mobility are important factors in creating the conditions for role reversal. The much improved level of living of the aged due to increases in the Social Security, medical insurance, and private pensions has made the phenomena of extreme old age dependence less likely than before. The current attacks on these programs may reverse the trend.

Not only are the improvements in the lives of many elderly resulting in a more satisfactory long life, but the recent political activity over concern with social security and media coverage of the needs and problems of the handicapped and disabled has indirectly helped them. Both the disabled of whatever age and the elderly have been denied access to jobs, status, and physical mobility accorded others in our society. Our medical advances and social welfare programs have given us many long-living disabled and normally endowed elderly. Since long life is the lot of most disabled people too, these problems and ultimate solutions are another consequence of long life.

Physical decline and disabilities of aging are difficult to accept in a society that places great emphasis on growth and productivity. Adding fifteen or twenty years to the average lifetime, and considerably more for a substantial number, may help to bring about a more sophisticated view of the implications of growth and productivity. The simplistic assumption that growth is the only alternative to death or stagnation is being seriously questioned.[64] Baltes, a psychologist, has stated, "growth is not the only legitimate development concept."[65] New thoughtways that redefine and question the idea that the essence of life primarily involves growth and productivity could have a substantial impact in making the prospect of long life satisfactory rather than apprehensive.

Long life requires that new norms, values, expectations, and ultimately new social organizations and institutions be developed in order to give the aged more control over their own lives. As present populations grow old, the number of people with chronic disease and disabilities of various kinds will increase. More people will live in residential settings designed for the very old, in which independence and control are sharply curtailed. The conduct of service providers and the organization and management of old age residences will have to be developed so that there is as much self-determination as possible for the elderly residents. The prevalent assumption that the aged normally revert to child-like behavior at an indeterminate advanced age is untenable.

If the aged who are not in the labor force are to be given the chance to live out their lives as fully as possible, society will have to be structured to provide the prerequisites for the maintenance of self-esteem and self-control. This implies a considerable change in the "aging establishment."

It may be arguable that the large number of aged and the awareness of the importance of self-control can affect a change in relationships between those who need help and those who do the helping. As such, one consequence of long life will be social changes that increase the potential for a better life during the last years of the life course.

REFERENCES AND NOTES

1. Ariès, Phillipe: *Centuries of Childhood: A Social of Family Life.* Translated by: Robert Baldick. New York, Knopf, 1962, pp. 38ff.
2. Peter Berger in the New York *Times,* March 20, 1969, C13.
3. Johnson, Elizabeth S.: Older mothers' perceptions of their child's divorce. *The Gerontologist, 21*: 395-401, 1981.
4. Hareven, Tamara: The lost stage: historical adulthood and old age. *Daedalus, 105*:18, 1976.
5. Hill, Reuben: Decision making and the family life cycle. In Shanas, E. and Streib, G. (Eds.): *Social Structure and the Family: Generational Relations.* Englewood Cliffs, N.J., Prentice-Hall, 1965.
6. Hughes, Everett C.: Cycles, turning points and careers. In Hughes, Evertt C. (Ed.) *The Sociological Eye.* Chicago, Aldine-Altherton, Vol. I, 1971, pp. 124-131.
7. Neugarten, Bernice L.: The awareness of middle age. In Neurgarten, Bernice L.: (Ed.): *Middle Age and Aging.* Chicago, University of Chicago Press, 1968, p. 98.
8. Butler, R.N. and Lewis, M.I.: *Aging and Mental Health.* St. Louis, C.V. Mosby, 1977, p. 138.
9. Neugarten, B.L. and Hagestad, H.: Age and the life course. In Binstock, R. and Shanas, E. (Eds.): *Handbook of Aging and the Social Sciences.* New York, Van Nostrand, 1976, p. 45.
10. Neugarten, B.L.: Continuities and discontinuities of psychological issues in adult life. *Human Development, 12*:125, 1969.
11. Demos, John: Old age in early New England. In Demos, John and Boocock, S.P. (Eds.): *Turning Points: Historical Sociological Essays on the Family. American*

Journal of Sociology, 84: Supplement, 1978, p. S262.

12. *Ibid.,* p. S263.
13. U.S. Department of Health and Human Services. Public Health Service: *National Estimates of Marriage Dissolution and Survivorship: United States.* Hyattsville, Md., National Center for Health Statistics, 1980, p. 17.
14. Pumer, Morton: *To the Good Long Life.* New York, Universe Books, 1974, p. 12.
15. Hess, Beth B. and Markson, Elizabeth W.: *Aging and Old Age: An Introduction to Social Gerontology.* New York, Macmillan, 1980, p. 265.
16. *Ibid.,* p. 266.
17. Helsing, Knut, Szklo, Moyses, Constock, George W.: Factors Associated with Mortality after Widowhood. In *American Journal of Public Health, 71 (8):* 802-809, 1981.
18. New York *Times,* July 13, 1981, p. A10.
19. Miller, Stephen J.: The social dilemma of the aging leisure participant. In Neugarten Bernice L. (Ed.): *Middle Age and Aging,* Chicago, University of Chicago Press, 1968, p. 371.
20. *Ibid.,* p. 372.
21. Shott, Susan: Emotion and social life: A symbolic interactionist analysis. *American Journal of Sociology, 84 (6):* 1331, 1979.
22. *Ibid.,* p. 373.
23. Fried, Edrita: Attitudes of the older population groups toward activity and inactivity. *Journal of Gerontology, 4:*1969, 141-151.
24. Rosow, Irving: Adjustment of the normal aged in Williams, *op. cit.,* p. 210.
25. Blau, Zena Smith: Changes in status and age identification. *American Sociological Review, 21:*201, 1956.
26. *Ibid.,* p. 202.
27. Lowenthal, Marjorie Fiske and Haven, Clayton: Interaction and adaptation: intimacy as a critical variable in Neugarten, *op. cit.,* 1968, pp. 390-400.
28. Neugarten, Bernice L.: The future and the young. *The Gerontologist, 15(1):*9, 1975.
29. Rosenmayr, Leopold: Achievements, doubts, and prospects of the sociology of aging. *Human Development, 23:*54, 1980.
30. *Ibid.,* p. 54-55.
31. Parsons, Talcott: Socioculture's pressures and expectations. In Simon, Alexander and Epstein, Leon S. (Eds.): *Aging in Modern Society,* Washington, D.C., American Psychiatric Association, 1968, p. 37.
32. Labouvie-Vief, Gisela: Adaptive dimensions of adult cognition. In Datan, Nancy and Lohmann, Nancy (Eds.), *Transitions to Aging.* New York, Academic, 1980, p. 12.
33. Kline, Chrysee: The socialization process of women: implications for a theory of successful aging. *The Gerontologist, 15(6):*492, 1975.
34. Rose, Arnold M.: *Theory and method in the social sciences.* Minneapolis, University of Minnesota, 1954, pp. 50-71.
35. Atchley, Robert C.: *The Social Forces in Later Life: An Introduction to Social Gerontology.* Belmont, Calif.: Wadsworth, 1980, pp. 338-339.
36. Tamir, Lois M.: *Communication and the Aging Process: Interaction Throughout the Life Cycle.* N.Y., Pergamon, 1979, p. 96.

37. Robert C. Peck, "Psychological Developments in the Second Half of Life," in Bernice L. Neugarten (Ed.), *Middle Age and Aging: A Reader in Social Psychology,* Chicago: University of Chicago, 1968, p. 91.
38. H.A. de Vries, *Report on Jogging and Exercise for Older Men,* Washington, D.C.: Administration on Aging, Department of Health, Education and Welfare, 1968.
39. Palmore, Erdman: Sociological aspects of aging. In Busse, Ewald W. and Pfeiffer, Eric (Eds.): *Behavior and Adaptation in Late Life,* Boston, Little Brown and Co., 1969, p. 49.
40. Bulter, Robert N.: The facade of chronological age: An interpretive summary. In Neurgarten, *op. cit.,* 1968, p. 242.
41. Wantz, Molly S. and Gay, John E.: *The Aging Process: A Health Perspective.* Cambridge, Mass., Winthrop, 1981, p. 138.
42. Lubinski, Rosemary B.: Why so little interest in whether or not old people talk: a review of recent research on verbal communication among the elderly. *International Journal of Aging and Human Development, 9(3):*241, 1978-79.
43. Sheppard, Harold L. and Rix, Sara E.: *The Graying of Working America: The Coming Crisis is Retirement Age Policy.* New York, Free Press, 1977, p. 67.
44. Beauvoir, Simone de: *The Coming of Age.* New York, G.P. Putnam, 1972.
45. Ward, Russell A.: *The Aging Experience.* N.Y., Lippincott, 1979, p. 46.
46. Butler, Robert N. and Lewis, Myrna I.: *Aging and Mental Health,* 2nd edition. St. Louis, C.V. Mosby, 1977, pp. 284-85.
47. Resnik, H.P.L. (Ed.): *Suicidal Behavior: Diagnosis and Management.* Boston, Little, Brown, 1968. Seiden, R.H.: Mellowing with age: factors influencing the nonwhite suicide rate. Paper presented at the 13th annual meeting, American Association of Suicideology, 1980.
48. Bock, E. Wilbur: Aging and suicide: the significance of marital, kinship, and alternative relations. *Family Coordinator. 21(1):*71-8, 1972.
49. *Ibid.,* p. 75.
50. Sainsbury, P.: *Suicide in London.* 1955, p. 81.
51. Kruijt, Cornelis S.: Suicide: a sociological and statistical investigation. *Sociologia Neerlandica. 3:*44-56, 1965-66.
52. *Ibid.,* p. 53.
53. Riley, Matilda W. and Foner, Anne.: *Aging and Society.* Volume 1, *An Inventory of Research Findings.* New York, Russell Sage, 1968, p. 363.
54. Maas, H.S. and Kuypers, J.A.: *From Thirty to Seventy.* San Francisco, Josse-Bass, 1974.
55. Setlin, Joan M. Some thoughts on diseases presented as senility. *The Gerontologist, 18:*71-72, 1978.
56. Gutmans, D., Grunes, J., and Griffin, B.: The clinical psychology of later life. In Datan, Nancy and Lohman, Nancy (Eds.). *Transitions in Aging.* New York: Academic Press, 1980, p. 120.
57. *Ibid.,* p. 120.
58. Parent, Mary K. The nature of stress in middle age. A paper presented at the Gerontological Society annual meeting in Dallas, Texas, November 20, 1978, p. 2.
59. *Ibid.,* p. 2.

60. *Ibid.,* p. 2.
61. *Ibid.,* p. 3.
62. Glasser, Paul and Glasser, Lois.: Role reversal and conflict between aged parents and children. *Marriage and Family Living, 24*:46-51, 1962.
63. Lowenthal, Martin: The social economy in the urban working class. In Gappert, Rose (Ed.) *The Social Economy of Cities.* Russell Sage, 1975, 447-546.
64. Schumaker, Sale and numerous others are included.
65. Rosenwayr, *op. cit.,* p. 57.

Chapter 5

LONGEVITY AND SOCIAL ASPECTS
OF AGING

THE scientific study of aging is a relatively new development. An aspect of the history of aging is expressed in the many attempts to delineate the various phases of human life. The early classifications provide a backdrop for modern attempts to determine the beginnings of old age. Ancient Chinese scholars divided life into seven phases:[1]

Youth	to 20	yrs.	of	age
Age for contracting marriage	" 30	"	"	"
Age for performing public duties	" 40	"	"	"
Learning one's faults	" 50	"	"	"
Final period of creative life	" 60	"	"	"
The longed-for age	" 70	"	"	"
Old age	From 70 yrs. of age			

Rosset aptly concludes that the longed-for age, constituting the ages from sixty to seventy, was rare and hence "longed for."

Pythagoras, in the sixth century B.C., made the course of human life analogous to the seasons. He proposed a sequence of life beginning with spring, the period from infancy to youth (0-20 years); youth represented summer (20-40); full adulthood corresponded to fall (40-60 years); and the winter of life was old age and retirement (60-80 years).[2] The two ancient definitions of old age, based on the stages of the life course, encompass the most common range of years currently used in defining old age, sixty to seventy.[3] This is primarily a demographic definition based on the probability of death with implicit references to biological changes.

Biologists are moving towards a scientific explanation of life and death, but have been unable to develop an acceptable theory of the aging process.[4] There seems to be agreement, however, that aging occurs at varying rates in human beings. Unlike the biological features of infancy, youth, and maturity, there are no universal functional or structural changes that allow a definite boundary to be drawn between middle and old age. The organs of the body deteriorate at varying rates. Stresses and strains of the biological, psychological, and social environment have such important consequences for the human organism that a strictly physical-chemical explanation of aging is of limited use.[5] The natural lifespan has also been difficult to identify due to the lack of knowledge regarding the precise nature of the aging process.

Although genetic factors play a role in determining senescence and death, many gerontologists believe that "individual differences in longevity are more a function of environmental differences than of inborn potential."[6] We are still in that period of human history when control of environmental factors, such as the diseases of midlife, nutrition, and psychological stresses, are the basic factors in determining length of life.

Aging in the biological and social psychological sense varies tremendously. Biologically, we move toward senescence by fits and starts. "Progress toward old age resembles . . . the descent of a staircase rather than the continuous movement of an object gliding down an inclined plane."[7] The sequence of maturational phases occurring from infancy to adulthood move upward from one plateau to another. This appears to be similar to the decline from middle age to death.

Within the context of social roles in modern society, role expectations for specific age levels vary from one part of society to another. Since the great increase in numbers of old people is of recent origin, the definitions of old age behavior have not yet become clear-cut. Long life and affluence for many people creates a fluid situation. The norms for the old are as much in flux as are those for the young and more active members of modern industrial society.

Our cultural milieu provides us with the definitions and expectations for the way we should act and when in relation to our chronological age. As we have noted, these expectations have little relation to the individual's abilities or desires. Society defines the appropriate behavior for each age-group: "for the individual, the awareness of age expectations becomes an important basis for his own self-perception; for the society, age-group expectations form a basis for the allocation of social roles."[8]

Social and psychological aspects of aging appear more variable than biological aging. This has resulted in a lack of symmetry between the various processes of aging. For example, the present-day conceptions of the ideal life course seem at variance with the fact that physical deterioration begins to be clearly perceptible at the halfway mark. This lack of symmetry, between the ideal and the real, is heightened by our veneration of youth and the high status of youthful types of behavior. The anxiety stimulated behavior of men and women who spend fortunes on cosmetics, beauty spas, and health camps and emulate youthful behavior by extramarital sex and other exploits connoting youthfulness are some of the consequences of the lack of symmetry.

The disparity between the social and biological dimensions of aging generates a wide range of attitudes toward life. The range will be broadened as the perception of the near certainty of old age becomes more common. The capacity to deal with this expanded horizon and the lack of clear societal guidelines for handling it seems to be related to the peculiarities of "personal biography."[9] Our capacity to successfully negotiate role changes, sorrows, triumphs, and the many unexpected consequences of long life in modern society is closely related to our previous performance in handling the demands of life. In contrast to the step-by-step mode of biological aging, advancing age in social and psychological terms seems unsystematic and fluid.

The lack of a systematic and readily definable point at which old age occurs is further confounded by the absence of change in certain aspects of one's self-conception throughout much of life. Feelings, attitudes, and values may change very little over the span of years from youth to old age. It is quite clear that

> most people over seventy are secretly young, disguised in old skin. The aging and the old don't think of themselves as aging and old and don't see themselves as others do. It may take an aging woman much longer to wake up in the morning and come away with a result that satisfies her. An aging man may find, among other things, that his clothes no longer fit as well. Both sexes would rather not have too many mirrors around. But underneath that aging skin and body, both may feel as alive as ever, and with a strong need to celebrate life. Unfortunately, custom and tradition say they're not supposed to: when they do show feeling, they're likely to get startled, strange, or outright hostile looks from younger people. So they usually hide it, retreat behind their skins, and go into the limbo of "being

old"[10]

This concerns many who are approaching old age.

With greater longevity, the concern about aging increases. This is partly a consequence of the awareness that the definition of being old is highly variable and imprecisely defined. Variability in the definition of old is partly due to the improved levels of health and well-being, as well as the heterogeneity of occupations and life-styles that characterize modern society.

Beginning at approximately age forty, the process of physical aging begins to become evident for most individuals. Psychologically, we are confronted by the physical facts of age, but in terms of careers, jobs, education for job advancement, or divorce and remarriage, forty is still an age when a considerable amount of choice is possible.

Concern with loss of hair, excess fat, exercise, and health foods are not new vanities, but the belief that incapacity and death may be postponed by following certain kinds of activities and restraints is new. This recent awareness stems from the widened dissemination of scientific knowledge to the common man, especially from biology, nutrition, and medicine. New perceptions are shaping a fresh perspective regarding such questions as "When am I old?"

In an historical period when the speed of technological change has reached an unprecedented level, we also must cope with a monumental change in the duration of life itself. This fact makes it difficult to unravel the causes and consequences that are related to longevity. As has been argued here, however, the consequences are of primary and ultimately far-reaching nature.

Viewing these changes on a worldwide basis reveals considerable unevenness in the relationship between longevity and technology. Wilbert Moore poses a typology of societies in discussing the communication gap faced by the aging numbers of various societies.[11]

Traditional society marks the first type. In such societies, social change is relatively slow, and each succeeding generation is able to share the time-tested procedures and practices of the past. The roles and life-styles available are limited and tend to be repeated from one generation to the next.

The second type embodies more rapid social change. Under such circumstances, the older members of society must plan and expend effort in catching up on the innovations that take place over short periods of time. The emergence of all types of refresher courses and the recognition that obsolescence can be applied to humans as well as machines are evidence of this kind of society.

Type three describes a society in which the changes are so rapid that the aged and those of late middle age are often forced out of the competitive struggle. The mounting tempo of change puts the younger productive members of society in the top positions, and involuntary retirement and middle-aged unemployment become manifestations of this type of changing society.

The fourth type is one in which the rapidity of change has accelerated to such an extent that not only do the elderly become obsolete, but individuals in their late thirties and forties find themselves lacking the newest skills and perceptions required by the impelling nature of science and technology and the social responses demanded by continuous change. Within this type of society, large segments of both young and old find themselves out of step, and obsolescence ceases to be a function of longevity and aging. Moore asserts that the most advanced industrial societies come under this category.

Longevity has a wide variety of consequences depending upon the type of society in which it takes place. In traditional society, the extensions of living time has least effect, although it will probably have important consequences. The mere fact that death during the early and productive years becomes less common can have important effects for any society over the long run. In addition to this is the concommitant decreased depletion of each birth cohort.

The prolongation of life has meant that societies throughout the world include increasing numbers of aged people. The social problems of the aged did not come into existence until the early part of the twentieth century. There was an absence of the problem in earlier times because the few who did get old had a definable place in the social structure. The elderly were not segregated in the same way as modern retirees, since many of them worked to avoid the alms house or poor farm.

The problematic aspects of great numbers of aged persons spurred societal action into adding such programs as Old Age Assistance and Social Security. Germany was the first country to enact a compulsory old age assistance program in 1889; Great Britain followed in 1925. The United States was relatively late in dealing with the economics of an aging population. The Social Security Act was enacted in 1935. Thirty years later, in 1965, the U.S. Congress recognized the severe medical problems of millions of old people and enacted the Medicare program.

Friedman has stated that our concern for the aged has had an important effect in defining society's concern and obligations for the individual.[12] This has resulted in the formation of the values and institutions appropriate to a welfare state. It would be difficult to establish specific causal connections between concern for the aged and any general increase in society's obligations to the individual. It is, however, apparent that this concern is a major addition to the earlier societal concerns relating to education, hazards of unemployment, minimum wage, establishment of public recreational areas, and so on. Thus, longevity has contributed a new dimension to citizenship and complicated the growing functions of government.

As noted previously, early scholars exhibited great interest in cataloging the various phases of life. This was done, although relatively few lived to experience a third to a half of the possible stages. As the importance of a large aging population increased and the science of social gerontology developed, it became possible to categorize the social dimensions of aging more accurately.[13] As said before, the chronological ages of sixty, sixty-five, and seventy have been the most widely used numbers for the beginning of old age, but studies that have focused on *middle* age rather than on *old* age have shown that the turning point comes much earlier in adult life.[14] In fact, increased longevity has probably contributed more to the importance of middle age and later maturity than it has to old age when defined as occurring in the sixth and seventh decade. It is in the age of the forty's and fifty's, that the prolongation of life has had and will have the greatest social conseqences. Being stimulated to deal with long life during middle age increases our capacity for ordering or reordering our lives in order to live more fully to the end.

Old age has provided many contemporary men and women with an unprecedented amount of uncommitted time. The development of the ability and the perspective needed to use the time adequately must begin in middle age or earlier. Long life requires that socialization for old age begins long before old age takes place. Middle age may allow extra free time from the reduction of family and work responsibilities; this change can provide time and energy for making plans as well as changes in goals and behavior that are functional for an approaching later maturity and old age.

The Elderly and Social Change

The idea that age brings on rigidity and conservatism in attitudes and values is a common conception that accompanies the growing awareness of the aged in modern society. Though social scientists are progressing towards unraveling the factors that relate age and social change, the oversimplified explanation for such complex phenomenon as attitude change will not disappear easily.

It seems clear that as the elderly find themselves losing status and economic position conservatism and hostility to such change might occur. Hostility would be a rational response to real and threatening events, since a considerable portion of the social changes that have occurred in the drive toward modern industrial society have had disruptive effects on the status of aged populations.

Cottrell has compared the place of the aged in high and low energy societies. In a general sense, ". . . the emergence of high energy technology had been accompanied by weakening of the elements of the social structure upon which the aged had in the past relied to secure their ends. The new emphasis upon the market and other economic institutions, while it made the system more technically competent to provide an increased flow of goods, provided no certain way by which the aged could claim a share of that increase or even to guarantee to them the economic goods and services which they were able to enjoy in low energy society."[15]

It was found in a study done in Italy that the lower the economic level of the community was, the higher the status of the aged in the family. "The more impoverished the economic structure, when the existence of each individual is rendered precarious from outside the family, the scanty resources of old people (the ownership of the house, their modest pensions and the hard-earned produce of land) take on a special importance and, with them, so do the old people themselves."[16]

In contrast, as the opportunities for employment increase outside of agriculture, the young find work elsewhere, though they often live at home on the farm with elderly parents. Thus, the work experience and life-style of the older generation come to lack direct relevance to the new and emerging work — and life-style of the young.

In a transitional area in Holland, the social position of the aged changed in a manner similar to that studied in Italy. The apparent frustrations experienced by the young adult generation due to the limits of work available in agriculture and the restrictions of the extended family have threatened and decreased the power and prestige of the older generation. A manifestation of this is seen in some farmhouses that were being remodeled into two separate living quarters, "although still under one roof the younger and older generation now lead lives of their own."[17] Since the high social position of the aged in the community was based on their power and prestige in the extended family, the adoption of the nuclear family by the middle generation has resulted in a decrease in the position of the elderly.

Social change of this nature, as experienced and interpreted in areas of transition such as Italy and Holland, is highly conducive to the apparent development of rigidity and conservatism on the part of the aged. There is also evidence that older adults possess a concern for the maintenance of stability in the social order. They may therefore be seen as conventional. Some refer to this as rigidity, when in fact, it is adaptive and to the advantage of society.[18]

Kooy writes that "for generations, the problem of old age was primarily biological; today it is often social and cultural."[19] He perceives that the elemental feature of recent social changes is comprised of the growing individualism that manifests itself in the nuclear family and the changes in work rules. In turn, he accounts for the individuality of the Dutch family by pointing to ". . . Social Darwinism; romantic love; economic stratification; greater purchasing power; more extensive internal migration; larger cities; 'massification' (the inability of people to realize traditional goals and maintain moral standards because of conflicting social opportunities); social mobility; better educational facilities; changing social controls; and declining church attendance."[20] When extensive social change takes place, there is a high probability that it will appear threatening to many segments of the population, and hostility may occur. Such hostility, however, that seems to occur among the aged will usually only continue as long as the changes affect them negatively. "When change affects the entire society and tends to be assumed as a major cultural value of the whole population, the attitudes of older groups undergo substantial modification. Elderly people do not become alienated from society."[21]

An increase in the development of individualism is one of the important changes that has occurred in modern society. Whatever losses have been sustained by the aged due to increased individualism may ultimately be balanced by an expansion of opportunities for both young and old. Freedom of choice that can accompany individuality could help to make the last fifteen to twenty years of life a better time for the elderly than in the past. This will be discussed further in subsequent chapters.

The type of reflections on the past that are engaged in by the aged may have a positive effect on the attitude of the old towards social change. As a by-product of individuality, reflection on the past pertains to one's judgment of the level of success or failure that has characterized one's earlier life. Justification or rationalization for perceived failure often emerges from such reflection on personal history. In a study of residents in an old-age home, Pagani found that the residents often made unsolicited and insistent remarks regarding the improvements that had occurred in economic conditions at the time, differing from their own youth and early adulthood.[22] The residents made efforts to justify their present economic and social position by claiming that conditions in the past had made success much more difficult to achieve. As such, their attitudes were closely related to their attempts to maintain some kind of acceptable level of self-esteem.[23] When the benefits of industrialization have not been somewhat equitably distributed among the entire population, a variety of both conservative and radical attitudes will be generated under transitory social conditions.

The necessity of justifying one's major work role after retirement may be an inevitable component of the aging process. However, the degree of importance that this reflective activity takes varies with our capacity to choose our major roles and to change them voluntarily throughout life. Most societies seem to be structured in ways that put a temporary premium on inflexibility and denigrate change or vacillation in role choice. The young man who chooses his life's work early and singlemindedly pursues his goal follows the desired model.

However commendable such singleminded goal-striving may be for the first two-thirds of one's life, it may result in a rigid approach to the last third. Bennett Berger has commented on this issue indirectly in a discussion of a contemporary criticism of bureaucracy, organization men, and other-directedness. Though he wrote in response to Friedenberg's *Vanishing Adolescent,* it has as much relevance for late middle age as it does for adolescence:

> . . . I am not quite convinced that the bureaucratic virtues such as imper-
> sonality, adaptability, flexibility, and other-directedness are as unam-
> biguously inhuman as Friedenberg seems to think. Certainly adaptability
> may seem like spinelessness, flexibility like duplicity, and other-
> directedness like characterlessness, but a firm identity often manifests
> itself as pigheaded, stubborn rigidity, and a clear, stable ego-identity
> might well become an intolerable burden in a rapidly changing society
> where social and geographic mobility puts enormous pressures on larger
> and larger numbers of people who must anticipate the new demands that
> unfamiliar life situations will make on them tomorrow. In a too neglected
> article some years ago, Daniel Lerner . . . had the temerity to suggest that
> the real significance of the apparent spread of other-directedness might
> well be that a net increase in the imaginative and projective capacities of
> the population was occurring; that, indeed, other-directedness required an
> inordinate talent for role taking, which is of course, at root an imaginative
> talent, a sensitivity to others.[24]

In another context, Robert Butler deplores the fate of elderly men whose earlier lives have been maladaptive due to ignorance, rigidity, and missed opportunities. He writes of the truncated nature of human lives:

> When one listens to the old tell their lives, one senses . . . that most human
> behavior is maladaptive. No one tells the child that his life is the one and
> only life he has, that it must he carefully nurtured, that it is easy to 'blow it'
> . . . No one helps prepare him to be resilient (not malleable), resourceful,
> and proactive, by proactive is meant initiatory. The sources of action and
> decision could be in the self. Yet one's behavior need not be forecast and
> traced out with an indelible pencil. Nontheless, given the inequalities and
> failure of education, most lives have been wasteful in comparison to what
> could be.[25]

Butler considers the response to life of most people as rigid and involving "enforced identity." These responses to unsatisfactory roles are in the form of lives that have an infrastructure. Sometimes they are manifested in secret or hidden activities, as in the case of the weekend hippie, participants in group sex, or the extra-marital affair. Others live barren and cheerless lives by continuing to do work that is hated, but maintained for the sake of status and income.[26] Several other types of *infra-lives* are characterized by those who lead "lives of quiet desperation." Some are included among the 10,000 or so middle-aged people who disappear annually in the United States.[27]

Longevity, coupled with an acceleration of technological and social change, makes the commentary of Berger and Butler very pertinent. The prolongation of life has had and will continue to have important consequences in terms of new roles, individual identities, and the rigidity of behaviors imposed by society. In transition to a longer life, such obvious new roles as retiree, member of a postparental family (after children have left home), or emeritus member of a profession will become common roles. They may even have a temporal duration that exceeds that of some major work roles.[28] As these role changes become expected and as increasing numbers of people join the ranks of the aged throughout the world, new roles will become institutionalized; there is a great potential for wide variability in the way these roles can be played.

A great number of older people in the population are available, in a sense, for natural experimentation and innovation in learning how to live out a long life. For example, a degree of acceptance for early retirement to a life of leisure, old age marriage, old age sexuality, and old age travel has developed in recent time.

Despite the changes in acceptability of some of the new roles of the elderly, the aged are often singled out as especially problematic in a changing society. In contrast, the apparent rigidity, conservatism, and reactionary behavior of some of the middle-aged and youthful segments of the population are ignored. Social scientists, however, are becoming increasingly aware of the complexities underlying attitude formation and change. The findings and commentary of scholars and scientists imply that "There is no simple relation between age and attitude toward social change. We are again confronted with the necessity of elaborating different interpretations for different relations to various aspects of change. There is a strong suggestion that we need to revise the traditional idea that elderly people are culturally removed from the present and are hostile to change."[29] This is supported by the research literature on violent change resulting from disasters such as floods.

It was found that elderly flood victims were better able to cope with material and emotional losses than young victims. The competence of the elderly "in dealing with large scale disaster was so striking that the authors suggested that a support network of elderly females and males be organized to cope with future incidents such as floods and other natural disasters."[30]

Role Loss in Aging: Permanent or Temporary

Much has been written about the apparent loss of roles and normlessness that accompanies the aging process. This places the elderly in a social position that is undefined and ambiguous, a frustrating and difficult position to hold.[31] The norms of behavior that are generally required are few and ill defined. They encompass the norms of maintaining a residence separate from their children, keeping up social relations with children, and generally deferring to the middle-aged. A few general restrictions are also imposed on the elderly: behaving in a way commensurate with advanced age, doing the best to take care of oneself, and demanding the least possible assistance from helpers or caretakers, be they family or others.[32]

The lack of norms and the role losses of the aged are thought to stem from several causes, disengagement among them. It is the notion that aging inevitably leads to an ordered opting out of middle-aged activities and roles.[33] Roles are given up or lost, which is normal at earlier ages. It is, however, the failure to find new replacement roles that makes aging unique. The lack of social pressure or expectations for the development of new roles creates a perception of loss. The actual loss, or change from highly valued middle age roles, also contributes to the negative evaluation of old age. Tamir points out that "as long as the older individual does not behave too strangely, and as long as he doesn't lean too heavily upon those who provide for his needs, for the first time in adulthood he is allowed to say and do what he pleases. Only such factors as poor health or poverty can keep the old person from behaving precisely as he wishes. In other words, old people are allowed to be eccentric."[34] This should probably be qualified to state, "behaving precisely as one wishes," without serious penalty.

Unfortunately the right to do as one pleases is more a tolerance than a right and often accompanies low status. Children, youth, servants, and slaves are given the right to behave in idiosyncratic and deviant ways at least part of the time. That some aged people are found in the same situation fits their apparent loss of status. It is also conceivable that this freedom is an aspect of the perception of aging held by the middle-class middle-aged, who as a group may be at the peak of the life course, but are also somewhat coerced and constrained in terms of expectations and obligations.

The loss of roles and the failure to find new ones of sufficient social reward have been viewed as a consequence of the lack of role models. Rosow states that old age requires socialization to a "distinctive new role, new expectation and norms appropriate to it, and a set of eligible role models."[35] Since the number of elderly has been small in the past, especially those over seventy, an adequate number of live role models was impossible. Roles are not developed by a few isolated individuals (in age), but by large groups of peers and kin group members. Only among substantial numbers of peers, with similar histories and background, can new and experimental ways of behaving be tried with sufficient force to result in new modes of behavior. The number of aged are now sufficient for groups of them to forge new roles and standards of behavior for themselves and claim a larger place in the social order.

The increased length of life, which results in a slowdown in the depletion of the older cohorts, provides the larger numbers needed for the development of role models. In the past, the development of new role models for the elderly was almost impossible since death destroyed the necessary population base for their emergence. With the change in the timing of death, a new perspective and new lifestyle have contributed to the formation of new roles for the aged.

At present, one can discern the embryonic outlines of new roles, ones that vary on factors such as class, occupation, and ethnic group membership. For members of the white-collar middle class, roles for the elderly probably include increased travel for leisure and reestablishing kin group ties, commitment to volunteer work for a portion of time, change of employment sometimes resulting in second careers, and expanded leisure activity. Only paid work and leisured travel add much by way of status. At present, the emerging roles, whatever final form they may take, are not highly valued.

There is no doubt as to the loss of roles and status among many contemporary elderly. They have been subjected to the same kind of age-grading that has been visited on children and adolescents, a categorizing that tends to result in serious constraints. For the retired elderly, the result has been virtual institutionalization of a denigrated place in the social order.

In a partial sense, this is true for the reason given by Rosow. His reasoning is based on the way social class and prestige operate in the United States. "We value and reward people mainly in accordance with their *economic utility*. A person's social class position and relative prestige are ultimately anchored in the occupational structure, which makes social standing largely dependent on work roles . . . From this standpoint, the aged are severely disadvantaged, especially after retirement, and economic and technological changes are penalizing them further. For the pace of change accelerates the rate at which increasing segments of successive generation become economically obsolete and unessential."[36]

Although Rosow's description has a certain validity, it also contains some implicit assumptions that are questionable. He assumes that ecomonic utility is and will remain so strong a criterion that everyone bows before it. The status system is not monolithic. The heterogeniety in backgrounds and variability of life-styles and occupations in modern society have created a wide variety of status criteria for judging the worth of individuals and families. Different periods in the life course seem to vary in the assignment of status to activities, personal qualities, and possessions.

In youth and early adulthood, the status values assigned to athletic prowess, modern clothes, sports or customized cars, center city apartments, graduate school, and group behavior involving experimental use of liquor, drugs, sex, and car and auto racing may give added prestige to those who can afford to stake the right claims. Although many of these behaviors are rejected by the middle-aged population, they comprise a significant part of the overall status and class system.

For the middle-aged for example, occupational success, a high level of consumption, accomplished children, family activities including appropriate vacations, and social participation with prestigeful groups are paramount values. In turn, it seems that the elderly place increased value on creature comforts, financial stability, health, mobility, and independence. Although the class or economic component of these status criteria and symbols of prestige are important, a number of them are far from having a direct relationship to income and occupation. The factors of income and occupation, along with education, have contributed a great deal to the oversimplification of modern stratification systems. This is because income, occupation, and education are relatively easy to measure, and data is readily available on a large scale.

It is assumed that the elderly and late middle-aged, are somehow unable to respond to premature obsolescence by education or retraining. It also seems questionable to assume that our society will continue to allow large numbers of its productive members to slip out of the work force and become dependent on the productivity of others. The belief that the aging population is inherently incapable of learning is held by few, if any, gerontologists.[37] The assumption that our society will allow such losses of productivity can be questioned in light of the debate surrounding the financial problems of Social Security funding. The proposal to raise the retirement age for social security may become law in the near future. The new cohorts moving into the ranks of the elderly are much more educated and have been quite responsive to social and economic change that took place during their early and midlife years. This alone will force us to reevaluate questions of obsolesence and adaptability among the aging.

This view of the prospects for the elderly in modern society is in sharp contrast to Rosow's solution to the rolelessness of the aged. His solution would result in large geographic concentrations of aged in order for them to form their own subsociety or culture.[38] Presently, we do find a few concentrations of elderly, namely in Florida and Arizona, but this is a relatively small proportion of the older population. In fact, to bring together a large number of aged of similar social class, life-style, ethnic identity, past experience, etc., would be almost impossible, especially under conditions that would serve to insulate them from the rest of society. Any movement that occurs in this direction, by accident or design, would increase the prospects for obsolescence and inhibit the learning of new attitudes, norms, and skills. Added to that, the variety found among the elderly may preclude any policy that sought to bring them together. Neugarten found "that there is a wide variation in life styles among older people, enormous diversity, and multiple patterns of successful aging. There is no single pattern of disengagement, and no single or model pattern that produces life satisfaction. These findings apply not only to the younger aged — those in their sixties — but also to persons in their seventies."[39] In one sense, the presence of large numbers of elderly of the same age and the great diversity among them could speed the development of new norms and roles.

From our perspective, it appears as though Rosow's well developed thesis regarding the causes and consequences of role loss among the elderly suffers from its place in the history of social gerontology. The study of aging has been largely confined to cohorts of aged persons who form a bridge between the "old old" and the "new old." Kaplan has distinguished between important cohorts of contemporary elderly:

> There is a difference between what may be termed the "old old" and the "new old." It is more than an arbitrary year — such as eighty — within the segment of the elderly. Rather, it is an historical difference. The "old old" are those who, regardless of chronological age, were born and raised abroad. The major migration wave to the U.S. took place in the thirty years before World War I. Those who arrived about 1910 and were twenty years old are now (1979) eighty-nine. True, there are only 1.9 million persons over eighty-five in the U.S.A., but it is to them that much welfare was directed (they were in their 40s during the Depression); it was in their generation that legislation arose that moved us ultimately toward Social Security, OAO (Office of Aging) and the gerontological profession.[40]

The new old were born in the United States and are roughly in the fifty-five to sixty-five year age range. The youngest of them grew up benefitting greatly from modern biology and medicine. They also matured in an era of increased freedom, deciding the course of their lives. A part of this freedom, as we have argued, results from long life, and the accompanying new chronology of death and its social and demographic consequences. The new old represent a distinctly new kind of elderly population both in number and experiential background.

Leisure, Aging, and Longevity

The increase in leisure time in modern society has largely resulted from high economic productivity, the concomitant shortening of the work week, and the prolongation of life. Kreps has calculated that the American workers have gained about 1,200 hours of free, nonworking time per year over their 1890 counterparts. This increase is apportioned annually by a reduction in the workweek, an increased number of paid holidays as well as vacation days, and sick leave time. "In addition to a shortened work year, nonworking years have grown by about nine for a male at birth, with present life and worklife expectancies."[41] Those nine nonwork years can be credited to long life and an extension of the period of education. The gains in free time have affected primarily all those who have traditionally viewed work as the sine qua non of life itself.

Since earliest times, the rich and well born have had life-styles in which leisure was preeminent. There is a long tradition of abhorrence and avoidance of work among the nobility and upper classes of Europe. The privileged have generally conceived of little or no relationship between leisure and work. This is expressed in the observation that, among some segments of the upper classes, inherited or old wealth is accorded higher prestige than new wealth, which is gained by working. The increased length of life and shortening of the workweek have had little effect on the patterns of leisure of upper class life-styles.

In contrast, the relationship between work and leisure is changing substantially among the working people of industrialized societies. The increased free time has seriously affected the traditional ethic of work. For much of our social history, beginning long before industrialization, the Prostestant ethic has dominated the work-a-day life of the majority of men, women, and children. As an ethic that placed work close to Godliness, leisure could only be legitimated by being made important in improving the quality of work. As a result, leisure became viewed as *recreation*. An occasional respite from work could be justified if it resulted in greater efficiency and satisfaction. Leisure was, therefore, only fully justified if it enhanced one's productivity. For the middle and working classes, leisure for its own sake was not a legitimate way to spend large amounts of time.

Max Kaplan, an authority on modern leisure, has shown that contemporary views of the connection between work and leisure are in transition.[42] Workers in modern society, whose forefathers had been guided by the ethic of work, have begun to abandon the earlier views. They are affected by what Kaplan calls the new freedoms of industrialization, urbanization, unionization, and secularization.[43] With collective bargaining, the bulk of industrial workers gradually gained higher incomes and more free time. This results in a situation in which leisure is no longer subordinate to work.[44]

Kaplan has used the concept of *bulk time*, that is, free time arranged in longer lengths, such as long weekends, vacations, and retirement. The five-day week, instituted by Henry Ford in 1926, initiated the two-day weekend. This made new approaches to leisure possible. The relationship between work and leisure has been changing ever since. In Kaplan's recent work he writes, "With the car, the highway, the football bowls, and the TV specials comes also a growing ease with time in bulk. And bulk time feeds an upper-class ideology. It makes no difference whether the worker is blue or white-collar. The urge for leisure is color, class, and collar-blind. These days, on an individualistic and democratic level, the term to use and the process to watch is *life-style*. Here, too, we put our finger on leisure itself as a new social role — the heart of the potential meaning of retirement."[45] Nevertheless, those cohorts who are presently retired are a product of earlier times when the ethic of work was stronger. Many retired people feel impelled to introduce work-like aspects into their leisure time. The activity of these aged people must have a manifest goal that implies usefulness. "In much the same manner as the person preparing for an occupation attempts to determine the worth of the activity on which identity will be based, the aging retired person establishes the worth of his avocational activity to legitimize a base for a new social identity — that is, to justify a career of leisure."[46]

The continued trend toward long life for a larger proportion of the population is generating new definitions of leisure appropriate to long life. Predictably, these changes will increase the options open for leisure activity and continue to enhance the separation of leisure and work as distinct, though related, aspects of human life. The justification for leisure, in terms of improved productivity at work, is diminishing.

If, as Kaplan has stated, leisure is taking on a life of its own, some of the problems of the social acceptability of leisure activities will be alleviated among the retired and aged. However, de Grazia voices a pessimistic note in this regard: "(1) the absence of a strong cultural tradition of leisure; (2) a preoccupation with the accumulation of 'things,' and with wanting 'things' which cost money, work, and time and hence, lead to moonlighting, overtime, and a working wife rather than to the development of a tradition of leisure; and (3) the suspicion that leisure, that is, discretionary time utilized for self-fulfillment as distinct from off-work time, may be beyond the capacity of most people."[47] But the recreation industry is booming. More people in the United States are taking vacations, the arts and non-credit education courses are flourishing, and much of the mass media is dominated by sports programming. The evidence favors Kaplan's view rather than de Grazia's, and the increased awareness of the new chronology of life and death provides added incentives.

Leisure is increasing for everyone, but older people and youth have become major consumers. The potential of nearly full-time preoccupation with leisurely pursuits, particularly for elderly retired persons, has added a new dimension to social life. The suggestion has been made that a new profession of leisure counselors will emerge. These persons might be employed in factories, union offices, and in the executive suite. Their stocks in trade would be extensive knowledge of leisure activities and a theory for explaining the interrelationships of leisure to personality, work, family organization, economic security, and other conditioning factors and circumstances of life.[48] A number of professionals already perform some of the tasks relating to counseling or leisure, such as travel agents, social workers, psychiatrists, and editors of certain magazines and newspapers. Summer camp counselors, playground workers, and disc jockeys provide similar information and direction for the young. As length of life increases and particularly as the level of health of the elderly improves the need for knowledge and guidance along these lines will increase. This will continue until the uses of leisure during the whole of life become institutionalized in such a way that retirement to full-time leisure pursuits becomes an expected, planned, and fully integrated phase of the normal life course.

Longevity, Health, and Death

Illness and disease has social and psychological components that may have greater consequences than the physical aspect of a given disease. As Parsons has pointed out, illness is viewed as both "deviant behavior" and a somewhat legitimate "escape" from the competitive struggle that generates a fear of failure.[49] The use of illness in escape is of particular utility to the elderly. Since the aged are not expected to perform much of a useful function in society at present and are frequently viewed as objects to be cared for, the legitimacy of the sick role is enhanced. Being cared for in old age gives a "positive meaning to their place in the society."[50] Furthermore, the potentialities of the sick role are magnified under circumstances when there is a deficiency of socially important roles available for the aged. Despite the extension of life and the potential freedom to plan, change course, and enjoy new experiences, the lack of clearly defined expectations and desirable activities place a pall on old age.

Regarding the response of the aged to illness, Parsons writes ". . . why should a person recover from an illness or take good care of his health, if there is nothing worth while for him to live for? He cannot be 'forced to be free' unless freedom is the condition of something beyond it, which both he and the others whom he respects really want and value."[51]

Dubos has commented on the shifting characteristics of the heroes and heroines of literature relative to disease and death. The Romantic Period dictated that young, especially attractive, heroines suffer and die from some disease of langour, probably tuberculosis; the modern novelist gives his heroes and heroines the physical vigor and tanned complexion of well-endowed physical culturists; post-Romantic heroic models of popular fiction are being tempered by the so-called anti-hero, whose life frequently ends in violent death while he is a participant in a counterculture. Since many novels and the short stories primarily utilize characters who are young or middle-aged, evidence for a change in response to the awareness of long life may not be available from this type of cultural productivity.

In one sense, the rejection of contemporary culture during the 1960s and 1970s, as seen in the hippie phenomenon, may be interpreted as evidence of a change in acceptable life-styles. Some of these are not only contrary to current conceptions of the basic features of man's humanity and biology, but also ignore the cultural consequences of long life. The supposition that many successful men in the corporate worlds of business and government suffer from ulcers and premature heart disease and, in effect, commit suicide by following the so-called "bitch-goddess of success" increased the rejection of old norms and stimulated a search for new life-styles. Revulsion from a success-oriented, but foreshortened life, may be one aspect of the transition toward a longer, more varied life. Longevity means that life will become increasingly variable in type of occupational activity, status and prestige, physical capacity, and health.

Longevity has had great impact on the health sciences and the practice of medicine. The fact that men can now survive a long list of deadly infectious diseases to face an equally deadly set of chronic diseases has had enormous consequences. The proportion of persons over sixty-five who had one or more chronic diseases rose from 46 percent to 81 percent in the first half of the twentieth century.[52]

The nature of chronic diseases means that the cost in care and treatment of both living and dying for an aged person has greatly increased. This has provided the impetus needed for the adoption of national health programs throughout the industrialized world. It has even occurred in the United States, where the tremendous power of organized medicine has always been opposed to most governmental involvement. Ironically, as medical science improved its capability, the need for a more comprehensive approach to health emerged. Politics, law, and social science all became involved in the health field.

Among many social scientists, genetic causation is viewed as an anathema, though biology becomes important when dealing with longevity. It is apparent that as the average age at death goes up, all the varied genetic aspects of disease and aging gain importance. This is based on the fact that the length of time in which genetic factors can influence the organism is much greater for each individual. For example, if genetic factors play a role in such diseases as diabetes, cancer, arthritis, and certain heart diseases, the probability of contracting these diseases increases. Longer life provides more time for the effect of genetic factors to play out their role more fully. Consequently the importance of genetics in human life has increased with the prolongation of life.

Not only do the genetic factors that are related to specific diseases become more important, but the factors that are related to aging and deterioration itself take on new importance. Dealing with age-related disabilities is becoming a major concern to all those charged with the care and concern for the aged. If the new developments in genetic engineering are to reach a receptive audience and gain in potential, it will probably lie in the field of aging. Biological problems related to the loss of functions in sight and hearing and problems of physical mobility, which may or may not be genetically based, become important when large numbers live into the seventy's, eighty's, and ninety's. Though the lifespan itself may not increase appreciably in the near future, the need for improving the biological aspects of life during one's last years has become important. Already the increases in disabilities and diseases associated with aging has broadened the scope of medical research and practice. The terms geriatrics and gerontology have fully entered the vocabularies of the literate public.

Biological and medical science is beginning to establish a definite link between health and nutrition in old age. Although relatively little is known about the specific nutritional needs of the elderly, a number of diseases that occur in the later years appear to be linked to nutrition. Diet is important, not only by influencing the onset and severity of age-related diseases, but it may indeed also influence length of life.[53]

Based on the Ten-State Nutrition Survey (1968-70) by the U.S. Department of Health, Education, and Welfare, the major diet problems among the elderly involved obesity and starvation.[54] The findings indicated that although obesity is a problem, especially for women, many of the elderly do not get enough food of the proper variety. Nutritional deficiency is more prevalent among those over seventy.

Malnutrition among aged is the result of a lack of knowledge, as well as the social and psychological problems associated with personal losses that occur in old age. The losses of spouse, home, or physical mobility frequently affect appetites and interest in preparing meals. Joining these with decreased living standards, malnutrition is often the outcome. It is now apparent that malnutrition is a causal factor in mental illness. For example, dementia, which is an important problem among the elderly, seems to be associated with niacin deficiency.[55]

Although increased research is being done, relatively little is scientifically known about the *specific* nutritional needs of the elderly.[56] No nutritional standards are available for the sedentary elderly or those afflicted with common chronic diseases. Increased longevity has led directly to the acceleration of interest and research in this area of science. As a consequence of long life, age-related diets and nutrition will constitute a new and expanding area of important public knowledge in the immediate future. The large cohorts of the population, who are currently approaching middle age, are showing an increased concern with questions relating to health, nutrition, and exercise.

A recent development relating to medical science and long life poses the problem of handling the imminence of death among the aged as well as the many younger victims of terminal cancer or heart disease. In the past when death was frequent and apparently random in occurrence, mystical and irrational explanations flourished. With the control of disease, the decline of premature death, and the emergence of scientific explanation, the social acceptance of death as a nonmysterious and natural phenomena becomes a part of life perspective. Recently, attention has been focused on those who are kept biologically alive, but are mentally dead. The importance of this issue is seen in the recent congressional hearings on an attempt to legally define when death has occurred.

Dealing with the last days of certain widely publicized terminal cases has generated a surprising amount of literature in the past few years that is based on the new research interests of social gerontologists, social psychologists, physicians, and anthropologists.[57] The magnitude of known terminal cases, as well as the slow, lingering decline of many victims of these diseases, has inspired the development of special procedures and norms for handling death; the term *death management* has even been used.

The technical ability of the medical profession has given rise to questions about the impersonality and lack of dignity of death in the modern hospital. The use of tranquillizing drugs and the technical paraphernalia used in maintaining life are often applied to such an extent that the dying patient is socially and psychologically dispatched in a haze, surrounded by a multitude of tubes and machines in stark and sterile hospital rooms.[58] More frequently, the knowledgeable and perceptive elderly who are close to death wish to be free from the loneliness and the technical apparatus of the hospital.

To die with dignity is the concern of two organized groups in the United States.[59] To them, "indignity, . . . means deterioration, dependence and hopeless pain."[60] The public concern over prolonged dying has reached the point where a "right to die with dignity" bill has been introduced into the Florida state legislature. The bill would give a person that is suffering from an incurable disease the right to request that his or her life be ended.[61]

A modern movement based on an old idea has created the hospice.[62] It is a medieval term, referring to a place of refuge for the traveler. The travelers are those who are journeying on the road from the end of life to death. It has become apparent that dying people most need "relief from the distressing symptoms of their disease, the security of a caring environment, sustained expert care, and the assurance that they and their families won't be abandoned."[63] The specifically new organized facilities provide for the special needs of the dying by utilizing the skills of teams comprised of physicians, nurses, social workers, pharmacists, psychiatrists, and clergy. These special facilities for the dying were pioneered by Cicely Saunders in England and Elisabeth Kubler-Ross in the United States. They recognized that many of the terminally ill suffered a sociological death long before they actually died. Several terminal diseases inflicted such continuous debilitating pain that the end of life was often one of unspeakable misery. The hospice is very effective in making the process of dying much easier and infinitely more humane. It represents a highly enlightened and rational approach to death at a time in history when premature death has been greatly diminished. It is an important development in dealing with death in new ways under circumstances in which long life is the norm. Long life, with the resulting increase in degenerative diseases, has revitalized the old concept of hospice. It is an important modern medical institution. Though initially developed in England, hospices are now being established in the United States.

Longevity makes the early part of the lifespan relatively free from death only to make it frequent in old age. In the past, people were socialized to deal with death in the earlier part of the life course. Now that the timing and nature of death has greatly changed, we are developing new norms relating to death in old age.

REFERENCES AND NOTES

1. Rossett, Edward: *Aging Process of Population.* New York, The Macmillan Co., 1964, p. 89.
2. *Ibid.,* p. 90.
3. In pursuing their work in dealing with the aging of population, dependency ratios and the like, demographers have generally used the ages of 60 to 65 in developing their statistics, however, in the interest of a broader sociological sense, it seems more appropriate to extend the designation to age 70.
4. Rockstein, M., Chesky, J., and Sussman, M.,: Comparative biology and evolution of aging. In Finch, C.E. and Hayflick, L. (Eds.): *Handbook of the Biology of Aging.* New York, Van Nostrand, 1977, p. 28.

5. Birren, James E.: *The Psychology of Aging.* Englewood Cliffs, N.J., Prentice-Hall, 1964, p. 61; for example the rates of spontaneous death of cells, as well as the capacity for replacement vary widely from one organ of the human body to another.

6. *Ibid.,* p. 77.

7. Walker, Kenneth M.: *Living Your Later Years.* New York, Oxford University Press, 1954, p. 38.

8. Eisenstadt, S.N.: *From Generation to Generation.* Glencoe, Ill., Free Press, 1956, cited by Friedmann, Eugene A.: The impact of aging on the social structure. In Tibbitts C. (Ed.): *Handbook of Social Gerontology.* Chicago, University of Chicago Press, 1960, p. 120.

9. Thomae, Hans: Thematic analysis of aging. In Tibbits, Clark, and Donahue, Wilma (Eds.): *Social and Psychological Aspects of Aging.* (Proceedings of the Fifth Congress of the International Association of Gerontology.) New York, Columbia University Press, 1962, pp. 662-663.

10. Pumer, Morton: *To the Good Long Life: What We Know About Growing Old.* New York, Universe Books, 1974, pp. 7-8.

11. Moore, Wilbert: Aging and the social system. In McKinney, John C. and De Vyver, Frank T. (Eds.): *Aging and Social Policy,* New York, Appleton Century Crofts, 1966, pp. 39-40.

12. Friedmann, E.A.: The impact of aging on the social structure. In Tibbitts, *op. cit.,* p. 140.

13. Clark Tibbitts is credited with developing and popularizing the term in the 1940s, Streib, Gordon F. and Orbach, Harold L.: Aging. In Lazarsfeld, Paul F., Sewell, William H., and Wilensky, Harold L.: *The Uses of Sociology.* New York, Basic Books, 1967, p. 613.

14. Tibbitts, Clark: Origin, scope, and fields of social gerontology. In Tibbitts, *op. cit.,* p. 9.

15. Cottrell, Fred: The technological and societal basis of aging. In Tibbitts, Clark (Ed.): *Handbook of Social Gerontology.* Chicago, University of Chicago, 1960, p. 117.

16. Florea, Aurelia: The new status of old people in the family and their relationships. In Hansen, P. From (Ed.): *Age with a Future,* Philadelphia, F.A. Davis and Co., 1964, p. 456.

17. Kooy, Gerrit A.: Social system and the problem of aging. In Williams, Richard H., Tibbitts, Clark, and Donahue, Wilma, et al., (Eds.): *Processes of Aging: Social and Psychological Perspectives.* Vol. II, New York, Atherton Press, 1963, p. 53.

18. Labouvie-Vief, Gisela, Adaptive dimensions of adult cognition. In Datan, Nancy and Lohmann, Nancy: *Transitions of Aging.* New York, Academic Press, 1980, pp. 19-20.

19. *Ibid.,* p. 54.

20. *Ibid.,* p. 55.

21. Pagani, Angelo: The import of age on attitudes toward social change. In Williams, Tibbitts, and Donahue, *op. cit.,* p. 90.

22. *Ibid.,* p. 92.

23. *Ibid.*
24. Berger, Bennett: *Looking for America: Essays on Youth, Suburbia and Other American Obsessions.* Englewood Cliffs, New Jersey, Prentice-Hall, Inc. 1971, p. 4; reference to Lerner, Daniel: Comfort and fun; morality in a nice society. *American Scholar,* Spring, 1958.
25. Butler, Robert N.: Looking forward to what? *American Behavioral Scientist, 14:*125, 1970.
26. *Ibid.,* p. 125.
27. *Ibid.,* p. 126.
28. Kaplan, Max: *Leisure: Lifestyle and Lifespan: Perspectives for Gerontology.* Philadephia, W.B. Saunders, 1979, p. 19.
29. Pagani, *op. cit.,* pp. 99-100.
30. Giesen, C.B. and Datan, N.: The competent older woman. In Datan and Lohmann, *op. cit.,* p. 60.
31. Markson, E.W.: Disengagement theory revisited. *International Journal of Aging and Human Development, 6 (3):*183-86, 1975; Rosow, I., *Socialization to Old Age.* Berkeley, University of California Press, 1974.
32. Tamir, Lois M.: *Communication and the Aging Process.* New York, Pergamon, 1979, p. 105.
33. Cummings, E. and Henry, W.E.: *Growing Old.* New York, Basic Books, 1961.
34. Tamir, *op. cit.,* p. 105; Rosow, *op. cit.*
35. Rosow, *op. cit.,* p. 160.
36. *Ibid.,* pp. 152-53.
37. Schaie, K. Warner: Age changes in adult intelligence. In Woodruff, Diana S. and Birren, James E.: *Aging: Scientific Perspectives and Social Issues.* New York, Van Nostrand, 1975, pp. 111-24.
38. *Ibid.,* pp. 160 ff.
39. Neugarten, Bernice L.: The old and the young in modern societies. *American Behavioral Scientist, 14:*20-21, 1970.
40. Kaplan, 1979, *op. cit.,* p. 16.
41. Kreps, Juanita M.: Economics of retirement. In Busse, Ewald W., and Pfeiffer, Eric (Eds.): *Behavior and Adaptation in Late Life.* Boston, Little, Brown and Co., 1969, p. 85.
42. Kaplan, Max: The uses of leisure. In Tibbitts, Clark (Ed.): *Handbook of Social Gerontology.* Chicago, University of Chicago Press, 1960, p. 411.
43. Kaplan, Max: *Leisure, Lifestyle and Lifespan: Perspectives for Gerontology.* Philadephia: W.B. Saunders, 1979, p. 27.
44. *Ibid.*
45. Kaplan, 1979, *op. cit.,* p. 24.
46. Miller, Stephen J.: The social dilemma of the aging leisure participant. In Neugarten, Bernice L. (Ed.): *Middle Age and Aging: A Reader in Social Psychology.* Chicago, University of Chicago Press, 1968, p. 371.
47. Grazia, Sebastian de: *Of Time, Work and Leisure.* New York, 20th Century Fund, 19562, pp. 300 ff. and 369 ff.
48. Kaplan, 1979, *op. cit.,* p. 439.
49. Parsons, Talcott: Toward a healthy maturity. *Journal of Health and Human*

Behavior. 1:172. 1960.

50. *Ibid.*, p. 173. This point is also made by: Hayflick, Leonard: Prospects on human longevity. In Neugarten, B.L. and Havighurst, R.J. (Eds.): *Extending the Human Life Span: Social Policy and Social Ethics.* Committee on Human Development, University of Chicago, 1977, p. 9.

51. Dubos, René: *Mirage of Health.* Anchor Books, Garden City, N.Y., Doubleday & Co., 1959, p. 208.

52. *Statistical Bulletin,* New York, Metropolitan Life Insurance Company, August 1960, pp. 1-3; this data further serves to indicate the extent to which death was postponed for large numbers during the 55 year period. Being old in 1901 was quite different from being old in 1955.

53. Schaefer, Arnold E.: Nutritional problems of the elderly. *Nutritional News, 43(3):9,* 1980.

54. Harland, Barbara F.: FDA Regulatory concerns involving nutrition of the elderly. Speech given at the Gordon Research Conference, Colby-Sawyer College, New London, New Hampshire, July 29, 1980.

55. *Ibid.*

56. Watkin, Donald M.: Better nutrition for those already old: The challenge of the eighties. U.S. Department of Human Services: *Aging,* Number 311-312, Sept. and Oct. 1980, pp. 21-28.

57. New York University and Union Theological Seminary have offered courses on death, courses that were filled to capacity. *New York Times,* March 1, 1971, p. 35.

58. The maintenance of the bare minimum of life, in the case of the late President Eisenhower, for an extended period until final death has been publicly discussed and criticized.

59. Euthanasia Educational Fund and the Euthanasia Society of America.

60. The New York *Times.* March 1, 1971, p. 35.

61. *Ibid.*, p. 35.

62. Stoddard, Sandol, *The Hospice Movement: A Better Way of Caring for the Dying.* New York, Vintage, 1978.

63. Craven, Joan and Wald, Florence S.: Hospice care for dying patients. *American Journal of Nursing, 75(10):*1816, 1975.

Chapter 6

THE FAMILY AND LONG LIFE

"UNTIL death do us part" had a somewhat different meaning in the past. The disruption of marriage by death occurred so frequently and had such intense consequences that it seems incomprehensible when compared to contemporary family life. Changes in the prevalence of orphans, broken homes, stepparents, infant and childhood deaths, widowhood, emergence of new roles of postparental life, and the invention and development of life insurance have all had profound effects on family life. Let us examine the history of the family as it relates to the timing of death and the insights it provides on the impact of longevity.

Records from the seventeenth century show how the frequency of death affected the formation and duration of families prior to the modern age.[1] Laslett reports that in one community in England, approximately 25 percent of all marriages were not first marriages. Since divorce was illegal, this condition resulted from high death rates among adults. In the community of Manchester, over half the girls who were married for the first time were fatherless. A large proportion of brides and grooms came from the houses of stepmothers and stepfathers.

The literature of the seventeenth century contains many references to evil stepmothers and lonely widows, some of whom were thought to be witches. A local history reveals that in May of 1688 in Clayworth, England, 35 percent of all the children of the town were orphans.[2] They had lost at least one parent. Through most of the eighteenth and nineteenth century, the number of stepmothers and stepfathers had began to decline and eventually ceased being a prominent aspect of family life.

In Massachusetts, the number of women who died leaving orphaned children declined by 87 percent between 1830 and 1920.[3] During the last half century, a further dramatic decrease in the number of orphans has taken place. In 1920, one in every six children under seventeen in the U.S. had lost one or both parents, making an approximate total of 6.4 million children. By 1978, the number had dropped to 3.3 million or one in twenty. This decrease occurred, even though there were over three times as many children living in 1978 as in 1920. Most striking of all is the fact that the number of children who had lost both parents dropped from 750,000 in 1920 to 50,000 in 1978.[4] Five decades ago, orphanhood was a major problem, but orphanages have almost disappeared now. Various forms of public income-maintenance programs and other social services help to prevent the kind of family disorganization that was commonplace before the rise of modern urbanization and industrialization. These data clearly reflect the improvements in the longevity of the adult population, specifically mothers and fathers. Consequently, life for countless children has vastly improved.

The high marital mortality rates of the preindustrial age were accompanied by strong norms of remarriage. In a community in Yorkshire, England it was found that one man married his sixth wife in 1698 and a seventh in 1702. Although some American colonists lived longer than Europeans, remarriage was not only frequent, but came quickly after the death of a spouse. Frontier conditions were not conducive to long ceremonial mourning, a perspective that has extended itself to contemporary times. Calhoun vividly describes the practice: "Peter Sargent, a rich Boston merchant had three wives. His second had had two previous husbands. His third wife had lost one husband, and she survived Peter, and also her third husband, who had three wives. His father had four, the last three of whom were widows."[5] The succession of marriage and divorces that characterize certain groups in contemporary society have been called *serial monogamy*. The phenomenon is not new, but it is now divorce rather than death that has become the primary fragmentary agent.

From a number of European sources, the French historian Fourastié has provided data that reveal the profound changes that have occurred in the history of family life.[6] In the seventeenth and eighteenth centuries, the average marriage lasted fifteen to twenty years; by the middle of the twentieth century it had exceeded forty years. It has been estimated that French marriages will last an average of about forty-seven years during 1980-90.[7] These statistics emerge despite the fact that the age at marriage in recent times is only one or two years less than it was 250 years earlier.

The recent relative reduction in the rate of maternal deaths also has contributed to keeping the family intact. In 1900 for instance, married women in America aged twenty to twenty-four had a death rate 44 percent greater than that experienced by the unmarried of the same age.[8] Primarily as a result of the control of pueperal infection, the death of American mothers in childbirth declined from 600 per 100,000 lives in 1915 to 1 in 1977. Among whites alone, the rate was approximately 0.8 in 1977.[9] A number of European countries have an even better record.

A heroic, though ultimately tragic, episode in the life of I.P. Semmelwies (1818-1865) involved an attempt to prolong the life of mothers. He observed that of two obstetric clinics in Vienna, the one in which deliveries were done by midwives, differing from the one run by doctors and interns, had a markedly lower rate of puerperal mortality.[10] As had Oliver Wendell Holmes in the United States, Semmelwies concluded that the deadly infection was carried by the contaminated hands of medical men. He proved that a routine handwashing with a chlorine solution would result in a dramatic decline in maternal deaths. The rest of his short life was spent in sacrificing his mental and physical health trying to convince his contemporaries of the efficacy of his sterilizing procedure. That it took over three decades for such a simple act to become a part of obstetric procedures seems shocking to the contemporary mind.

It has generally been assumed that households in preindustrial times were large, resulting in extended families. After considerable historical investigation, Laslett concludes that such was not the case. He states that "no two married couples or more went to make up a family group; whether parents or children, brother and sister, employer and servants or married couples associated only for convenience. When a son got married he left the family of his parents and started a family of his own."[11]* In effect, the small nuclear family composed of father, mother, and children is not a new development at all.

Demographic research reveals that the extended family, with its elaborate vertical and horizontal organization, has been more ideal than real. In contrast to this ideal of the frontier, the family structure

From Peter Laslett, *The World We Have Lost*. Copyright © 1965 Peter Laslett (New York: Charles Scribner's Sons, 1965). Reprinted with the permission of Charles Scribner's Sons.

of nonliterate societies closely approximates the nuclear family of contemporary society in terms of size and the relationship of members.[12] This is especially interesting because the nuclear family has been considered the typical modern family type that has developed in response to urban life. High death rates, however, appear to have been the basis for the nuclear family in premodern times. The determining factors are somewhat different in present day urban society. Laslett further suggests that "the multigenerational family of kin living under the same roof or in close geographic proximity may even be somewhat commoner in the contemporary industrialized city than it was amongst the peasantry. Urbanization, mechanical communications, growth of wealth and the increase in expectation of life may actually have strengthened familial ties and widened the network of kinship."[13]

Research in England reveals that relatively few households contained in-laws in residence in the seventeenth century.[14] Furthermore, the occurrence of young married couples living with their parents after marriage was even more rare. Conversely, a couple seldom had aged parents living with them; generally the parents did not live long enough to make this necessary or possible.

Age of marriage and high death rates have an effect on the length of marriages and size of families. It generally has been assumed that our ancestors married much earlier than we do now, especially the women. Age at first marriage seems to have varied over time and from one place to the other. In fifteenth century Florence, age at marriage ranged from twenty-five to thirty-one years for men and eighteen to twenty-one for women. Epidemics like the plague and fears of overpopulation affected the age at marriage. Epidemics seem to have fostered an interest in marriage and childbearing:

> For patrician families, frequent marriages in the wake of epidemics doubtlessly sprang from conscious policy. The patricians desperately wanted male heirs (but not too many heirs); the death of a father or older married brother enabled — even required — younger males to marry, lest the lineage expire. But even among the less advantaged classes, massive deaths opened up numerous basic jobs and career opportunities, which gave to younger men the economic independence needed for marriage. Deadly epidemics, high mortalities, and shortened expectations of life consequently exerted downward pressures on the ages of first marriage, especially for men.[15]

Elizabethan brides and grooms averaged twenty-four and twenty-eight years of age at the time of marriage.[16] In contrast, American brides averaged twenty-one years of age and the bridegrooms twenty-three years in 1978.[17] There are records of early marriage, but they are confined to the wealthy, and apparently represent one of the concerns associated with money, privilege, and maintaining the family line. Since well-to-do families were few in number, their proportionate effect on the average age of marriage is small.

Since the formation of a new family unit had important consequences for the community with a subsistence economy, the time of marriage became a community matter. Before a marriage could take place in the European village culture of the preindustrialized age, a slot in the economic network had to be opened or created. In relatively stable subsistence economies, the possibility of creating new places depended on economic expansion, a condition that was infrequent prior to industrialization. Most couples, therefore, had to wait to be married until someone died or retired, raising the marriage age above what it is today.

Frequently, the short length of marriage inhibited fertility. A great variety of debilitating diseases and suckling each infant for a long time contributed to low fertility. In France, historical demographers found that fertility fell sharply for women in their late thirties, and ended completely at an earlier age than at present. It has been calculated that eight births per marriage was approximately maximum for the average marriage that had lasted through the full period of the wife's fertility.[18] According to data from the most studied areas of France, the peasantry averaged fewer than five births per marriage[19] towards the end of the century.

Social conditions that delay marriage, curtail fertility, and cause high death rates among infants and mothers have important consequences for social life and culture. Specifically, the length of life and the frequency of death affect the social relationships and roles that emerge within the family. The length and permanence of marriages are influenced by the timing of death.

Longevity and the Marriage Market

Long life can be socially characterized by the fact that it entail the successive abandonment of old roles and the adoption of new ones. A long family life together means that husband and wife experience the full gamut of role changes, beginning with youth or young adulthood and proceeding through the years of having preschool and young children, adolescents, launching period, young adults, postparental, and aging family.[20] For a couple, such a variety of role demands makes interpersonal and role conflict a preeminent condition of long life. The adaptability of each spouse to the demands of such a succession of roles will vary. While one is reasonably satisfied with life at the onset of the postparental period, for example, the other may find this stage of life difficult to accept. While sharing all of the small details of contemporary married life, the capacity for tolerance, affection, and intimacy is probably not equally distributed through the married population. For those of lesser tolerance, the longer the marriage lasts, the greater the likelihood of conflict leading to serious disenchantment with family life. On the other hand, modern marriage has been defined as primarily one of companionship.

One might hypothesize that at least three periods of the family cycle are the most likely to be periods of heightened companionship, the initial one being the first few years after marriage. The second is the postparental period, the third would comprise the last years of life when physical deterioration accelerates and the losses among age peers begin to escalate.[21] This implies that the child-rearing periods of the family life cycle are characterized by a decline in companionship. The difference between the roles of the mother and father seem greatest during this period, child rearing in the case of the mother and a nonfamily occupational role in the case of the father. The inability of coming to terms with the problems and circumstances of this long middle span of married life seems to be a major cause of divorce and separation.

As presently conceived, the family is a relatively limited social structure. To a great extent, its form is quite rigidly defined in an elaborate set of civil laws. The legalized rigidity of the family and the social norms defining acceptable behavior for adult members will continue to come under scrutiny and attack as a result of its perceived failures. Extended life has added as much as a quarter of a century in close living to many marriages. This, among other factors, exposes marriage to a phenomenal increase in disruptive influences and results in high divorce and separation rates. In effect, the decline of premature death has fostered the development of high rates of divorce and separation. With the new potential for a forty- to fifty-year average duration, the institution of marriage is in the throes of some substantial changes.

Change in the dynamics of the marriage market is closely related to the wealth of time possessed by the modern married couple. A few decades ago, the high maternal death rate gave the marriage market the fluid quality that now results from high divorce rates. A woman's marriage potential was related to the death rate, whereas it now has a closer relationship to the divorce rate. In the past, the women who failed to get married in the first round of marriages (that is, at the desired age) attained the matrimonial state in the second round due to the higher death rate of spouses.

It is probably safe to assume that monogamy will remain the basic form of marriage for some time to come, but for many it will be modified in terms of serial monogamy. Although first marriages may have a potential length of fifty years, many will not last that long. Currently, one in three marriages in the United States ends in divorce or separation. The high level of insight, good fortune, and highly adaptable personality required in a successful fifty year marriage is, as yet, not too plentiful among applicants for marriage licenses; hence, divorce and remarriage may increase in frequency, depending on age and rate of marriage.

With the emancipation of women, the burden of divorce is being lightened. Developing effective and economical day care centers for young children will give the single-parent family an added measure of freedom not possible at the present time. It will also allow a mother to enter the labor market with a minimum of inconvenience and concern. By avoiding confinement to the home, her chances for male companionship and remarriage are improved as well.

In the past, divorce threatened the future prospects for remarriage of women. However, the redefinition of middle and old age has relieved some of the hazards of separation and divorce. "We do not have to go back farther than the early years of the century to find a time when the average woman in her midforties was, by current standards, definitely 'old.' It was as if her childrearing function had virtually exhausted her capacities, and she had relatively little left to do. The preservation of feminine 'attractiveness' into much more advanced ages is an important symptom of a major change in this respect."[2] The change in attitude towards middle-aged women has been of considerable importance in facilitating remarriage. This is, of course, most important for divorced men and women, because widowhood now occurs much later than in the past. From 1900 to 1964, the median ages for widows rose from fifty-one to fifty-nine years, and for widowers from forty-eight to sixty-five. There may have been further increases during the past fifteen years.[23]

Like the policeman, mailman, or soldier who retires from one career and takes up another, increased longevity has facilitated divorce and remarriage. Two categories of divorced persons that have increased in recent years in the United State are couples who have young children and older couples who have been married for about twenty years.[24] This has had social consequences for many children.

As in the past, children may have to adapt to a new parent because of divorce rather than death. This has created a new set of family problems. For example, children must accommodate to dealing with a parent in two different homes. The conflicts of generation, family attachments, and emotional adjustment of growing up are increased in complexity by the new patterns of interaction imposed by divorce and remarriage.

Though longevity may have made divorce more common, other consequences of long life have contributed to the happiness of childhood. Essentially, the banishing of dangerous illness and death from childhood and the idealizing of one's early years as normally happy ones have transformed childhood. Peter Berger has even argued that the recent rebellion of youth results from one's "moving from the unbelievable happiness of childhood into confrontation with less bliss-producing social structures of the adult world."[25] The rapid change that has been taking place in the evolution of marriage and family is one such aspect of adult life that seems to be less than blissful.

For some people, marriage has become less important as a prerequisite for sharing a life together. For couples who do not plan to have children, marriage is not mandatory. The general relaxation of traditional sex norms and the redefinition of many social relationships have contributed to these changes. It is conceivable that we may be returning to a situation similar to that which existed in the medieval period, when an important reason for marriage was procreation. Child rearing, however, will probably continue to demand some kind of legally constituted and relatively permanent family structure for some time to come. Communal living has gained a degree of popularity and undoubtedly has a number of positive features associated with it, but it will not eliminate marriage, particularly for those couples who plan to have children.

With the advent of the contraceptive pill, new forms of sexual expression have become possible. The old prohibition, fear, and guilt associated with sex have been considerably reduced. However, the change has not led to a rampant promiscuity. "The personalism of postmodern youth requires that sexual expression occur in the context of a good relationship — of intimacy and mutuality. If the older morality that makes sexual expression outside marriage illicit has disappeared, it has been replaced by a new morality of 'meaningful relationships' — relationships in which, as one youth radical put it, 'people are good to each other.' "[26]

The scope of alternatives as to when, how many, and under what conditions to have children provide contemporary couples with a broader range of life-styles. The potentialities for varied styles of family life were quite restricted under high infant mortality, maternal mortality, and the premature death of fathers. Couples marrying at various ages may bear children at different points in the life course. From this, there emerges a variety of possibilities relative to family life-styles. For example, the problems and satisfactions of the postparental period for a couple who are highly educated and have had their children relatively late will vary substantially from a couple who are high school graduates, were married before age twenty, and had their children within three years of marriage.

The marriage success of families moving through the life course will be affected by the way in which they must meet the demands of successive historical events that impinge on family life. War, epidemics, prosperity, and depression can have profound effects. According to Irwin Deutscher, the Depression provided a type of socialization that was functional for postparental roles, though not exactly anticipated; it was effective socialization nonetheless. The 1930s may have fostered companionate marriage. In Deutscher's study of postparental life, he states

> The interviews are rich with tales of hardship and struggle, fought through together, with young children to care for. . . . Men, who had already nearly reached the top, found themselves suddenly unable to pay their utility bills. . . . One cannot be but impressed by the tremendous

resiliency of these middle class couples who, working together through what must have been great hardship and disillusionment, pulled themselves back up to their accustomed middle class level of living. All of them bear scars. Not unlike the ties that bind men who have served in the same combat units in wartime, these couples share something between themselves which not even their own children can fully understand. The Great Depression appears most certainly to have lent stability to these marriages and imparted a quality to the relationship of the spouses which serves them in good stead when they are thrust directly back upon each other after having children in the home for two decades.[27]

As discussed earlier, certain periods in the family lifespan may be more companionable than others, a condition that is attributable to the nature of the life course which has been influenced by longevity and social circumstances rather than the individual psychologies of the participants.

The Timing of Death and Family Organization

The impact of change on family organization that has been caused by a shift in the frequency and timing of death can best be seen by focusing on the roles of family members. From the social psychological viewpoint, roles represent patterns of attitudes, values, and expectations, and any change in the occurrence of death has social consequences for family roles. The consequences of death in the family have usually been studied with the aim of assessing the effects of the loss of a parent on the surviving children. The parental roles, however, are also modified by the death of children. Before the emergence of modern bacteriology and the subsequent development of immunization techniques, childhood diseases took a heavy toll, and the death of one or more children was almost always an inevitable aspect of parenthood.

An awareness of the high frequency of infant death provided strong motivation to have as many children as possible. As mentioned earlier, data from France prior to industialization showed that eight births was approximately the minimum number to ensure that a family would have offspring reaching adulthood. The attitudes toward young infants and children were conditioned by the possibility that a child would not reach maturity.

Ways in which the frequent occurrence of death affect the family are related to the consequences of death throughout the society. In the past, for instance, the use of myth, ritual, religion, and private discussion were all devices for dealing with the highly visible and ever present fact of death. Today, the discussion of death is often taboo. Conventional language patterns are filled with euphemisms for death, died, and so on. We use "passed," "passed on," "gone," "departed," "big C got him," and so on. Casual conversations turn to the weather, minor illnesses, or vacations, where formerly the conversation would frequently involve the sudden death of a friend or neighbor's child. Even for children, the socialization process in most modern countries no longer includes ways of dealing with frequent death. At one time, a child learned a repertoire of informal conversational styles relating to death and the formal norms of mourning, attendance at the death watch, funerals, and so on. In contrast, the young person of today suffers occasional embarrassment because he or she has never had the opportunity to learn or practice the traditional rhetoric appropriate in dealing with death. The great change in the timing of death has created a situation in which the psychological, social, and economic behaviors brought forth by death are mainly required in middle and old age. It is primarily in the socialization for the role of old age that the social and psychic preparation for death occurs.

During this century, the death rates for infants under one year declined from 164.4 in 1900 to 15.4 in 1976.[28] For the corresponding period, the rate for small children from one to four years was 19.8 and 0.8.[29] This decrease has diminished the possibility of a young person having any direct experience with death in the family or among friends until relatively late in life. Many now become middle-aged before they personally experience death in a way that has social and psychological consequences.

In contrast to the present, the prominent social historian, Phillipe Ariès, points out that during times of high infant mortality, the French did not recognize young infants as individuals in their own right. He states that "No one thought of keeping a picture of a child if that child had . . . died in infancy . . . it was thought that the little thing which had disappeared so soon in life was not worthy of remembrance. . . ."[30] "As late as the seventeenth century, in *Le Caquet de l'accouchée*, we have a neighbour, standing at the bedside of a woman who has just given birth, the mother of five 'little brats,' and calming her fears with these words: 'Before they are old enough to bother you, you will have lost half of them, or perhaps all of them'; a strange consolation: People could not allow themselves to become too attached to something that was regarded as a probable loss."[31]

The changes in mortality appear to have altered the status of the kinship group in modern society. For decades, social commentators have been heralding the demise of the family and the breakup of kinship groups. Social disintegration and the state of anomie were presumed to be the consequence. Although many of the predictions about the decline of the family are grossly in error, there have been distinct changes. Some of these are directly related to the new chronology of death. Increased life expectancy, decreases in the average age at marriage, and decreases in size of family have meant that the average child has some grandparents living for a large portion of youth and early adult life. For example, the average ten-year-old white child has the chance of having at least one living grandparent in nineteen out of twenty cases. Fifty years ago, the same child had only four out of five chances. Similarly, the opportunity of having at least two grandparents increased from two out of five, to approximately three out of four, in 1970. As might be expected, the chances of having a living grandmother are much greater than having a living grandfather. For a ten-year-old in 1970, the probability of having only one living grandfather was only one in fifteen.[32] At the very least, these data mean that the family has been broadened in scope by the postponement of death. As a result, the socialization of children is more likely to include interaction with old grandparents, and even with older great-grandparents. Succeeding generations of children will learn how to interact and appreciate those who are two and even three generations older than themselves. The experiencing of intimate social situations with older people may increase family solidarity and help improve attitudes toward aging.[33]

Many families will have one or more great-grandparents living and often in good health during the younger years of the children. This will mean a redefinition of the role of grandparents. In recent times, a considerable number of persons have become grandparents in their middle or late forties. Young grandparents generate a different set of roles from those that are appropriate for sixty- to seventy-year-old grandparents. A consequence of extended life may be that the great-grandparent roles will become more like traditional grandparent roles, with the result that present-day grandparent roles will lack clear definition. It is conceivable that youthful grandparents may become increasingly competitive with the parents in the rearing of children. However, a qualification is in order. Recent demographic data show a change towards lower birth rates and an increase in age at the time of marriage. This may signal a shift in future relative age differences between children and grandparents.

In estimating results of longevity on grandparent roles, it is more appropriate to concentrate on roles outside the extended family. It seems apparent that the problems of the aged and the lack of clearly defined roles can best be solved by looking to the community instead of the family. The development of alternative roles for the elderly that are functional for the community and neighborhood would lend stability to the role expectations of those who grow old. The usual grandparent-babysitter roles seem highly varied and unstable in modern industrial society. In effect, these roles in the family may diminish in importance.[34]

Longer life for all family members varies in its effect on the potentiality for kin-group relationships, especially during the later stages of life. During adulthood and the young-old years, it will be increasingly rare for a person not to have some family members alive. The resulting multigenerational families will, therefore, provide alternatives in family associational patterns. However, as the young-old cohorts age and reach the old-old stage (75 to 90 years) they will experience a loss of actual and potential kin-group relationships.[35] Some younger family members will themselves be in the young-old stage, hence less able to maintain relationships with the older family members; the young old may become infirm and even die, leaving the very old family members without their help.[36]

Although government programs ranging from Social Security, Medicare, and the Older Americans Act have given the elderly many needed support services, a whole new set of needs have emerged. These needs have resulted from the fragmented and bureaucratized nature of the support systems developed for families and the aged.[37] Middle-aged children are needed to provide guidance and counsel and even serve as advocates in order to ensure that the aged receive the benefits to which they are entitled. With the emergence of modern medical technology, the aged also need help in managing their own terminal illnesses. "Given the development of heroic efforts to sustain life, and the later ages at which old people face death, decisions must be made by the middle-aged offspring whether to continue or cease such efforts. There is an ironic symmetry here as the child supervises the parent's death in much the same setting as the parent gave life to the child. Although these decisions can bring renewed closeness to family members, they can also become occasions for displays of guilt and grief."[38]

This situation may be intensified in the future. Current population trends, resulting in a period of zero growth, will mean a low birth rate and an older age for motherhood. This will result in smaller kin-groups.[39] Smaller kin-groups will, in turn, mean potentially fewer family relationships for the very old. Moreover, the higher age at marriage and childbearing will separate the generations by more years, thus introducing the possibility of greater gaps between grandchild and grandparent generations.

The norms and behavior associated with zero growth and the fact of long life can be expected to result in more single old people due to lower marriage rates and increases in widowhood. With the prolongation of life, widowhood occurs at later ages. The potentiality for kin-group support that traditionally has been based on attitudes expressed by "blood is thicker than water" and "one must take care of one's own" will be weakened due to the larger numbers of aged who have no family. A cogent observation has been made about the potential loss of emotional and psychological support that is usually provided by the family; "in the absence of such a security blanket, perhaps individuals would feel compelled to hold vigorously onto their faculties and consequently live more self-actualized lives free of the many neuroses which are fostered by unchecked dependency."[40] A decrease in kin-group relations may elevate friendships in old age to a new level. "It is possible that the 'fictive-kin' relations, which have been observed within some low income black communities, may become more common in the future. Within these networks numerous longstanding friends are regarded as relatives, and strong expectations for sharing resources prevail."[41] Thereby, friends may become primary sources of companionship and emotional support. Neverless, despite the potential for new norms of friendship among the aged, the demographic changes resulting in the old-old being left without family support will require greater involvement of both business and government in adequately providing the services needed by the very old.

Postparental Life: New Roles for Men and Women

Nelson Foote worded it well when he wrote, "In one sense it is presumptuous to speak of new roles for men and women. The exploration of the infinite variety of relationships that are possible between two people of opposite sex has been going on since long before history began to be recorded."[42] In another sense, a great number of married couples have just begun to experience a postparental life. For the second time in their married life, a couple must now contemplate life without children in the household. ". . . Of the forty-two million married couples in the United States (in 1960), little more than half have children at home; of the childless couples, more than two-thirds are in the postparental category; that is, as many as fifteen million couples. And of these, most would consider themselves middle-aged, not aged."[43] The postparental period was rarely experienced in the average family until about 1900.[44]

The full significance of the changes made in 1900 is that only one or two generations are experiencing this new phase of life. This is historically unique in that such a large proportion of married couples are beginning to experience a postparental life, while an increasing number in an earlier birth cohort, are retiring from active work with marriages unbroken by death. Not only has the control over maternal death kept families whole, but the additional ability to prolong life has contributed to the development of an entirely new dimension of married life. In 1890, under the age structure existent at that time, the median age of the husband was fifty-seven at the time of his wife's death.[45] This catastrophe occurred on an average of over two years before his last child was married. In 1950, the husband's median age was sixty-four at the death of his wife, which occurred fourteen years after his last child had married (the difference is similar for the 1970s).[46] "The magnitude of this change can be appreciated if we consider that the post-child-rearing period for today's older couple is approximately two-thirds as long as the child-rearing period itself; and, for the individual, the male will spend approximately as much time and the female will spend 37 percent more time in the post-child-rearing period as the period of performance of their major family functions."[47]

The demographic factors that account for the emergence of postparental life are only partially the result of the decline of death rates during the child-rearing period and the general increase in longevity in middle age. Factors such as median age at first marriage, size of family, marriage rate, and age at birth of the last child are all integral parts of the combination of elements that make the new phase of life possible.

Since the postparental period is relatively "new," there are few clear-cut social expectations or norms governing what to do with it. That is, the roles of men and women have been drastically changed in marriage by the addition of more time in which to live together. New patterns of behavior are developing, and as they do, various groups and institutions of society will come to expect certain social behavior during the postparental period. This situation will force the development of a new set of roles in the lives of most married couples. The work of Bengtson and others indicated that the direct transmission of values from one generation to the next tends to be weak, and that considerable variability characterizes the value orientations of children, parents, and grandparents. Gaps in the transmission of values from one generation to the next indicate that new orientations and processes of socialization to postparental roles are continuously developing.[48] Although the added increment of living time affects the roles of father and mother primarily, an equally important consideration is the alteration that occurs in the husband-wife roles. Each of the two remaining members of the emptied nest are faced with a new and different set of adjustments.

During the adolescent years, the wife's behavior is dominated by her role as mother, even though she may be working outside the home. Although the husband's set of roles involves being a father, his occupational role is often more important. In many instances, work dominates the life of the husband. Most of his aspirations and energy are directed towards his work role. During the postparental period, the roles of husband and wife differ in that the husband's major role continues much as before, and the mother's role is sharply curtailed and permanently changed. It is marked by the onset of menopause and fewer child-rearing responsibilities. In contrast, the husband may well be at the peak of his career, reaching his highest income, and gaining the rewards of seniority.

The postparental period affects the wife and mother in much the same way that retirement affects the husband. Each must face a substantial change in their central roles, although the onset of the postparental period may precede the husband's retirement by ten to fifteen years.

With the recent developments in social gerontology, particularly in the United States, impetus has been given to consideration of the problems and role conflicts facing an aging population. The postparental period is one of the most important of the later ages of life, especially due to the fact that what happens at that point in life will have considerable impact on retirement and old age. The current problems of the postparental period stem from the fact that it is relatively new to our experience and that we are in transition relative to the roles that will ultimately become a part of family life. The older marital roles are inadequate, and there are few useful role models available; the development of an adequate socialization process is only beginning to emerge.

In dealing with the problem of role discontinuities and transition in family life, one researcher states that "In discussing postparental life, middle-aged spouses clearly reveal that it is not sound to assume that anticipatory socialization is absent simply because this is a new stage of the family cycle — that is, because middle-aged couples of today have not had the experience of observing their parents make such a transition."[49] He refers to a number of characteristics of American life that provide tangential, if not direct, anticipatory socialization. The veneration of change and the new for its own sake provides some social oil to smooth many of the changes demanded by a dynamic society. The pervasiveness of the mass media in sloganeering for change has become a permanent feature of our symbolic life. "You can't stand still," "If you don't grow, you're dead," "Progress is our business," and "Time for a change" are among the thousands of daily admonitions to adapt and change. Some people, particularly from the middle strata of society, have become accustomed to viewing their own lives as a process of successive changes. For them, the transition to postparental life is simplified.

Middle-class families frequently have the opportunity to experience the temporary absence of their children, while attending summer camps, visiting relatives, and going to college. A great many college-bound youth who have the choice prefer to continue their education away from home and thus contribute to making college an important element in the socialization of their parents as well as of themselves. Some conditions of work for both the middle- and the working-class strata can contribute to adult socialization. The man who travels frequently or has to live temporarily at a neighboring city in order to work at his trade begins the process of dissolving the family unit before the postparental stage. "If the work role helps to condition fathers for the departure of their children, at least some mothers appear to be provided with a conditioning device which is the distinctive property of their sex. That device is the cultural myth of the mother-in-law: 'As soon as my youngsters were born I made up may mind that I was not going to be a mother-in-law like you read about.' Such a resolution, if intended seriously, could go far in preparing a mother to accept the departure of her children."[50]

The demographic factors that shape the chronology of family life make the changes of postparental life most extreme for the woman. The early age at marriage, the closer spacing of children, and the decline in large families has resulted in median ages for family completion of twenty-six years for the mother and twenty-nine years for the father. Although as mentioned earlier, the active mother role, which the female parent generally never completed, has ceased to constitute a majority of the years a woman may spend in marriage. A significant characteristic of the maternal role involves a high degree of dependency on the husband. In earlier times, the average woman spent her entire life in a role that made her personally dependent upon others. Now the average woman may shed much of the dependent aspects of her feminine role at a relatively young age. At the age of forty-five, a substantial number of women have completed their parental roles. Statistically, they can expect to live another thirty to thirty-five years. A period of life of that length not only demands the adoption of new roles, but provides an opportunity for a considerable amount of choice.[51]

The added choice has meant a new freedom for the married woman. Since the exercise of choice generally demands planning as well as decision making, new responsibilities have also appeared. In terms of prevailing social norms, the new freedom of choice has provided a climate in which the sequence of roles for women has broadened beyond that which is available to men. The expectations for male behavior relative to family and occupational responsibilities are quite strong, but the additional living time for women and the transition to the establishment of new postparental roles opens up a wide range of choices.

Women's liberation movements have increased education for women. An already sizable minority of women in the labor force have also enhanced the openness of this period of cultural transition. In a sense, many of the women in modern countries have been given a second youth. Some of the same turmoil that is associated with the openness and fluidity of youth has occurred for women in the new postparental life. One of the broadest areas of choice is that of paid work. The most perceptible postparental role choices made by women have been those involving entry into the labor market. For many middle-class women, the transition to a role of gainful employment is made through some form of advanced education, be it technical or professional training.

In describing this transition, let us postulate a scenario for a middle-class woman. This woman goes to college, graduates, is married at age twenty-two, has two or three children, and spends fifteen years as a housewife and mother. She takes additional college work and by about age forty-one may even have earned a professional degree.[52] She begins working in her chosen field at age forty-five. Many women can plan for a second career of twenty to thirty years, depending upon their initiative and health. The noncollege or non-professional woman may have the opportunity of shopping from one job to another until she finds what suits her most. Along the way, she may gain the skills and proficiency needed to enhance the satisfaction derived from important and challenging work. Good health and an awareness of long life may stimulate a more effective search for satisfying work.

It is obvious that one of the motivations for middle-class women to work is the desire for income, but there is evidence that noneconomic reasons for entering the labor force are also of substantial importance. Middle-aged women entering the area of paid occupations substitute occupational achievement for that which has been traditionally associated with homemaking. Such a development implies that an expansion in new opportunities for achievement will be necessary in order to satisfy the demands of women in establishing postparental roles. Furthermore, "the increasing concern of middle-age women with occupational performance runs counter to middle-age male inclinations toward deemphasizing such performance. This could be a significant source of middle-age marital conflict."[53] The full impact of the woman's new postparental role in an achievement-oriented labor market is difficult to predict at this time. A change in the definition of marriage roles, age of entry into the labor market, and the future of education for women will all influence the social outcome of the phenomenon of the middle-aged working wife.

The history of fertility in the United States supports the contention that bearing children has been one of the prime roles of women. That function, and the basic elements of the role it calls forth, probably qualify as the most institutionalized activity of women. Decline in the infant mortality rates and the acceptability and effectiveness of new methods of contraception have spurred on a new rational approach to family planning. It is partially responsible for the feasibility of early marriage. Youthful marriages become more acceptable when effective birth control methods are readily available. The new developments in contraceptive devices provide for more accurate family planning. Control over infant mortality and the high survival of all children allows a degree of freedom in family decision making that has never been possible before. Since women of the industrialized parts of the world mature earlier with menarche occurring at an average age of 12.8 years in the United States and menopause at age fifty, there is additional time for childbearing. The life course of women under contemporary circumstances provides additional time for making choices. It will be a long time, however, before men and women everywhere fully perceive their lives in terms of such a range of choices. A growing awareness of this may be seen in the current development of women's rights movements.

In terms of women's roles, the control of death from infectious disease, particularly those that killed infants and children, has done more to liberate women than any other single set of developments. A planned number of children evenly spaced and concentrated within four or five years during early married life, economic affluence, an emphasis on individuality, and long life forms a solid basis for the liberation of women. It is within the context of longevity and the lengthening of middle age that a substantial part of the life-scenario will be developed for the liberated woman. Any real change in the status of women implies socialization for the exercise of individual rights, beginning in childhood; nevertheless, it is the high probability of long life and the perspective it generates that serves as the backdrop, as well as the stimulus, for equal rights for women. Women's potentialities come into sharp relief when it becomes apparent that the average couple can have a married life of thirty to forty-five years. In addition to that, less than half of the women's adult life will be spent in bearing and rearing her children, if she chooses to have any at all.[54]

Not only has the control of death given married women a potential choice of new roles, but it almost guarantees that every mother may become a mother-in-law and a grandmother and quite likely a great-grandmother.

The postponement of death has given the role of mother-in-law a prominent place in the lives of middle-aged women. In years past, the duration of this role was usually short. The in-law role, which the humorist has belabored so often, is frequently the focal point of conflict within families. Both in-laws and grandparents can play an important part in widening or bridging the so-called generation gap, depending upon the adaptability and life perspective of the adults involved.

The active parental roles diminish relatively early and new roles take their place, but the relationship between parents and their children generally do not end until death. Although it is the duration of the parental role that has changed dramatically, the nature of the role has also changed, and a cluster of new roles have been added. As the roles of family members emerge, an alteration occurs in the social, economic, and psychological relations between children and parents.

Long life brings parents and middle-aged children together in new ways. As mentioned earlier, the middle-aged child will find it increasingly necessary to become involved with aged parents as guide and protector. Although this role may be intense and problematic and require considerable time, it differs from the past. It has been pointed out that present day postparental couples belong to

the first cohort of offspring who are fully released from an obligation to provide at least a minimum level of income maintenance and health care to their parents. Conversely, the aged parents are aware that they need not depend upon their children for their basic subsistence. Hess and Waring (1978) contend that intergenerational relationships are in the process of redefinition from obligatory to voluntary, and that what may look to some as a collapse of family bonds, could more accurately be considered a strengthening. When ties of affection and caring are maintained from a mutual wish to do so, they are deeper and more satisfying than when sustained out of duty or necessity. But this is not to say that parent-child relationships in later life will be free of controversy or sacrifice.[55]

For example, the circumstances of an incapacitated parent may require a decision on the alternatives of living in the home of the middle-aged child or in a nursing home. If a family takes in the ailing parent, the result may be a strain on time, energy, and financial resources, whereas the nursing home alternative may lead to guilt and ill will.

Although parents who live for a long time may pose problems relating to the independence of their children, adjustment to the in-law roles, and the health of aging parents, the parental home can provide great support in meeting many of the problems and hardships of early adult life. The familiar face and locus of one's childhood and adolescence can offer solace in the case of broken marriages, problems with children, occupational defeat, or the tragedy of premature death. Parental aid for education, travel, and the down payment on a house is becoming the sine qua non of proper middle-class parents during the early years of short budgets. The expected support function of the middle-class American family seems, at times, to have reached extraordinary proportions. In 1971, a New York family court ordered a father to continue the financial support of his daughter's hippie life-style by paying her college tuition and living allowances, though he strenuously disapproved of her activities.[56]

As significant changes occur in the roles of women, some changes will necessarily occur in the roles of men. At this time, the extended life of males has served to make retirement from the labor market a major event in the later years. It was unusual, in the recent past, for a man to stop working voluntarily. Now, such a change in the male role has become expected, regulated, legislated, and provided with all kinds of prescriptions for insuring a successful change. Longevity has lengthened the career of the male and added more years of retirement. However, for an increasing minority, the extended life has made it possible to plan an initial career and a career-like avocation or two careers. Many of those who enter the police force, the military, professional athletics, and some of the other professions officially retire from their initial career while in their forties or fifties.

Most of these men pursue second careers.

Long life demands more planning than was necessary in the past, when the average man died with his boots on. In order to insure a satisfactory retirement or second career, planning must take place before the actual event occurs. Purchasing annuities or life insurance or making arrangements for a second career for those who retire early all involve planning earlier in the life course. This fact gives life a different perspective from that which existed when life was shorter. A short life makes planning a frivolous pastime.

Long life is almost a certainty for many, though it will often involve widowhood. Many women and fewer men (every year twice as many become widows as widowers) will experience the role of widow or widower. Currently, the average woman has a life expectancy of almost eight years beyond the average man. For many, widowhood will last longer than a decade. The loss of a spouse represents such a serious role change that new knowledge, flexibility, and the willingness to initiate changes are required in order to make this part of life satisfactory. Long life has contributed to longer widowhood.[57] The new residential patterns that separate the generations in their housing arrangements require individual capabilities that were needed when the elderly widow was usually part of a younger family and widowhood lasted a shorter time. The present day needs of widows has spawned efforts to provide help through books, educational courses, counseling services, and social clubs.

Longevity cannot claim full credit for some of the newer aspects of social roles for family members. It is, however, the extra increment in living time of the average person that will affect family roles as the new features made possible by longevity become institutionalized. Long life allows a number of new activities to become part of the institution of the family, as well as the other insititutions: politics, economics, education, and religion. As yet, it is not fully apparent what these additions will constitute. Longevity, however, cannot be viewed as the cause, it is rather a necessary condition for certain changes to emerge.

Longevity and Life Insurance

The economic consequences of longer life and a sense of individualism were important factors in the rise and widespread use of life insurance. A large population, rational organization of labor and the accumulation of capital, and a productive agriculture provided the industrialization needed to raise the level of income for large modern societies. Personal incomes that were high enough to allow payment of regular premiums made insurance protection feasible. The ideology of individuality and self-reliance was instrumental in the development of attitudes and values favorable to life insurance in Britain and the United States.[58]

Life insurance originated in classical times and possibly earlier. The Romans used a form of endowment insurance. Roman Legionnaires were paid money in celebration of a victory, though they were required to deposit a part of it, which was either returned to them when they left the army or was paid to their relatives in the event of death. In the English speaking countries, the earliest recorded life insurance association was formed in England in 1699, the Society of Assurance for Widows and Orphans.[59] In 1705-6, an organization called the Amicable Society for a Perpetual Assurance office was formed, which was apparently the first permanently successful insurance company of England. Compared to modern methods, its practices seem not only strange, but unsound. In its early years, the Amicable Society deducted the expenses of conducting business from its income and divided the remainder among the beneficiaries of those who had died during the year.[60] In some years the benefits were generous, but sometimes they could be defined as meager and grossly unfair. It is noteworthy, that the origin of serious efforts in life insurance began in the early eighteenth century when the length of life was beginning to show a steady increase. Although unpredictable, natural disasters like famine and plague were still very much a feature of human life. The increased productivity of agriculture and the improvement in diet and sanitation began to push the curve of life expectancy upward.

This vital curve has been going up continuously on a worldwide basis. The data and methodology needed for a practical development of life insurance emerged in the nineteenth century.[61] At midcentury, John Graunt began the systematic analysis and publication of vital statistics based on the English Bills of Mortality. In the same period, Edmund Halley, the astronomer, constructed the first mortality table, called the Breslau Table, which gave the probable duration of life for each age. Life insurance was then possible.

Life insurance became a practical consideration for the average person when the expected age at death rose to a point where the annual premiums became small enough to make it economically possible.[62] There were substantial differences in the size of premiums on a life insurance policy calculated in 1840 and 1977. Data on the average remaining lifetime of men and women in 1840 and 1977 reveal that a cohort of males aged twenty in 1960 could expect to live seventeen years longer than an equivalent cohort in 1840. Women of the same age could expect to live twenty years longer in 1960.[63]

Life insurance ultimately rests on the norms and values involved in the balancing of risk and security by individual families.[64] Strong and extensive kinship systems and traditional village culture decrease the importance of insurance, whereas the intimate, urban nuclear family increases the risk involved in the loss of a single family member. A strong kin-group structure might minimize the importance of insurance were it not for the norms supporting the preeminence of the kin-group in protecting the family against disaster. It is conceivable that a strong kin-group system could equally well develop norms demanding a relatively high level of insurance protection for its members.

A factor in the develoment of life insurance was the full emergence of the intimate nuclear urban family. The new conceptions of individual choice in mate selection plus an increase in family social isolation led to a heightened level of intimacy in the nuclear family. The lessening of kinship ties and the increase in family isolation began with the enclosure movement in the seventeenth century. It continued with the mass Atlantic migration and is now ending with the rural to urban movement throughout the industrialized world. A social climate that fosters freedom of choice in marriage, geographic mobility, and the dissolution of extended family and community bonds proved to be fertile ground for the growth of individuality and self-reliance; a great many attendant political, economic, and religious ideologies nourished it as well. This kind of social milieu made possible a large-scale transformation in attitudes and values regarding the potentialities of human life. It gave the impetus to minimize the devastation of premature death in the family. Within a few years, insurance became the credo of responsible adults in the rising middle class. In place of burial insurance, established by the early fraternal organizations of American immigrants, came income assurance for the victims of a deceased breadwinner.

Longevity and economic affluence have resulted in the widespread purchase of life insurance, and they have had an impact on the shaping of certain family attitudes and values. The act of buying insurance forces the adult members of a family to think more rationally about death and its financial consequences. Values based on the maintenance of loose kin-group ties, i.e. those outside the immediate family, the ideal of intimacy, and the close emotional bonds of the modern family are all supported through the use of insurance. Planning to prevent the financial dependence of one's immediate family on the larger kin-group in the event of premature death helps maintain the ideal of self-reliance and freedom of choice. This ideal is a part of the ideology associated with choosing a mate and establishing an independent family. Despite an emerging shift toward the family, the ideology is still strong.[65]

Life insurance has helped raise the social and economic status of women. By reducing the hazards of the premature death of husband, father, and breadwinner, the wife and mother becomes less dependent.

Table 6-I shows the radical change in the economic strength of American families with regard to one of its greatest hazards. The average family is now protected by life insurance that is twice the amount of the annual disposable family income. In 1978, the average family had over 35,000 dollars in life insurance. Only eight countries in the world have life insurance levels that exceed average family incomes: Canada, United States, Sweden, New Zealand, The Netherlands, Japan, The United Kingdom, and Australia.[66] These are among the countries of the world that are most industrialized and have the highest life expectancies. The spectre of the alms house, the county farm, and the orphanage are all becoming a part of literary history.

An illustration of the importance of life insurance can be seen in the record of life insurance payments during the Great Depression. In the United States, payments of 15,600,000,000 dollars were made to insurance beneficiaries from 1933-1938. This amounts to three billion more than the Federal government spent for relief during the same period.[67] It is hard to escape the conclusion that the facts of human history surrounding the invention and development of the seemingly simple principle of spreading the risk has had an enormous impact on the future of family relationships. It is especially true since long life makes it possible for more people to participate throughout the world.

Table 6-I

Life Insurance and Disposable Personal Income
Per Family in the United States

Year	Life Insurance Per Family	Disposable Income Per Family
1930	$ 2,800	$ 1,900
1940	2,700	1,700
1950	4,600	4,100
1960	10,200	6,100
1970	20,700	10,100
1978	35,100	17,800

Source: American Council of Life Insurance, Life Insurance Fact Book, Washington, D.C., 1979.

REFERENCES AND NOTES

1. The following material on family and marriage in the seventeenth century is taken from Laslett, Peter: *The World We Have Lost.* London, Methunen & Co., 1965, p. 98ff.
2. *Ibid.,* p. 95-96.
3. Uhlenberg, Peter R.: A study of cohort life cycles: cohorts of native born Massachusetts women, 1830-1920. *Population Studies, 23*:414, 1969.
4. The data on orphans was taken from: Shudde, Louis O. and Epstein, Lenore A.: Orphanhood — a diminishing problem. *Social Security Bullentin, 18*:17, 1955, and U.S. Bureau of Census, *Statistical Abstract of the United States: 1979*:(100th ed.), Washington, D.C., 1979.
5. Calhoun, Arthur W.: *A Social History of the American Family From Colonial Times to the Present.* Vol. I. New York, Barnes and Noble, 1945, p. 70.
6. Fourastiè, Jean: De la vie traditionnelle a la vie "tentiaire." *Population, 14*:424, 1959.
7. *Ibid.,* p. 424.
8. Jacobson, Paul H.: *American Marriage and Divorce.* New York, Rinehart, 1959, p. 139.
9. U.S. Bureau of Census, *Statistical Abstract of the United States; 1956, 1979.* Washington, D.C., pp. 66; 75.
10. Ackerknecht, Erwin H.: *A Short History of Medicine.* New York, The Ronald Press, 1955, pp. 174-75.
11. Laslett, *op. cit.,* p. 90.
12. Coale, Ansley J., Fallers, Lloyd A., Levy, Jr., Marion, Schneider, David, and Tompkins, Silvan A.: *Aspects of the Analysis of Family Structure.* Princeton, Princeton University Press, 1965, pp. 49ff; 64-69.

13. Laslett, Peter: The History of Population and Social Structure, *International Social Science Journal, 17*:598, 1965.
14. Laslett, *op. cit.*, p. 90ff.
15. Herlihy, David: Deaths, marriages, births, and the Tuscan economy (ca. 1300-1550). In Lee, Ronald D. (Ed.): Population Patterns in the Past. New York, Academic Press, 1977, p. 151; the foregoing data on average age at marriage in Tuscany also comes from this source.
16. Laslett, 1965, *op. cit.*, p. 82.
17. U.S. Bureau of the Census, *Statistical Abstract of the United States: 1980.* 101st edition, Washington, D.C., 1980, p. 83
18. Laslett, 1965, *op. cit.*, p. 101.
19. *Ibid.*
20. This classification of stages of family life was developed by Hill, Ruben: Decision making and the family life cycle, In Neugarten, Bernice L.: *Middle Age and Aging.* Chicago, University of Chicago Press, 1968, p. 288.
21. Stinnett, Nick, Carter, Linda M., and Montgomery, James E.: Older persons; perception of their marriages. *Journal of Marriage and the Family, 34*:667-72, 1972.
22. Parsons, Talcott: Toward a healthy maturity. *Journal of Health and Human Behavior, 1*:170, 1960.
23. Riley, Matilda W. and Foner, Anne: *Aging and Society,* Vol. I, An Inventory of Research Findings. New York, Russel Sage, 1968, p. 165.
24. U.S. Department of Health, Education, and Welfare, Public Health Service, *Vital Statistics of the United States,* Vol. III, Marriage and Divorce. U.S. Gov't. Printing Office: Washington, D.C., 1964, 1965, 1966, 1967, 1968, p. 2-9.
25. The New York *Times,* March 26, 1969, C, 12.
26. Keniston, Kenneth: *Young Radicals: Notes on Committed Youth.* New York, Harcourt, Brace and World, 1968, p. 281.
27. Deutscher, Irwin: From parental to post-parental life: exploring expectations. *Sociological Symposium,* No. *3*:55, 1969.
28. U.S. Bureau of Census, *Statistical Abstract of the United States: 1971 and 1978.* Washington, D.C., pp. 56, 60, 70.
29. *Ibid.*, 1974, p. 60; that is, death for both sexes per 1,000 population based on midyear estimates, exclusive of stillbirths.
30. Ariès, Phillipe: *Centuries of Childhood: A Social History of Family Life.* Translated by Robert Baldick, New York, Knopf, 1962, p. 38.
31. *Ibid.*, p. 38, and *Le Caquet de l'accouchee,* 1622.
32. Metropolitan Life Insurance Co., *Statistical Bulletin,* September, 1972, pp. 8-10.
33. Bengtson, Vern L., Clander, Edward B., and Haddad, Anees A.: The "generation gap" and aging family members: toward a conceptual model, pp. 246-249, and Wood, V., and Robertson, Joan F.: The significance of grandparenthood, p. 286, both in Gubrium, Jaber F. (Ed.): *Time, Roles, and Self in Old Age.* New York, Human Sciences Press, 1976.
34. Back, Kurt: Personal characteristics and social behavior: theory and method in Binstock, Robert H. and Shanas, E. (Eds.): *Handbook of Aging and Social Science.* New York, Van Nostrand Reinhard Co., 1976, p. 425.
35. One large nursing home in Iowa has a population in which over 25 percent are

over 90 years of age, *The Daily Record,* Cedar Falls, Iowa, March 1980.

36. With advanced age (80 plus) choices involve more younger people than age mates, Bultena, Gordon L.: Age-grading in the social interaction of an elderly male population, In Bell, Bill D.: *Contemporary Social Gerontology.* Springfield, Ill., Charles C Thomas, Publisher, 1976, p. 246.

37. A whole book on family and bureaucracy has appeared: Shanas, E. and Sussman, M.S. (Eds.): *Family, Bureaucracy, and the Elderly.* Burham, N.C., Duke University Press, 1977.

38. Hess, Beth B. and Markson, Elizabeth W: *Aging and Old Age.* New York, Macmillan C., 1980, p. 266.

39. Shanas, Ethel and Hauser, Philip M.: Zero growth and the family life of older people. *Journal of Social Issues, 30:*85ff, 1974.

40. Williamson, John B., Evans, Linda, and Mumley, A.: *Aging and Society.* New York, Holt, Rinehart and Winston, 1980, p. 112.

41. *Ibid.,* 112, *see* Stack, Carol: *All Our Kin: Strategies for Survival in a Black Community.* New York, Harper and Row, 1974.

42. Foote, N.N.: New roles for men and women. *Marriage and Family Living, 23:*325, 1961.

43. *Ibid.,* p. 326.

44. Deutscher, Irwin: The quality of postparental life: definitions of the situation. *Marriage and Family Living, 26:*52, 1964.

45. Glick, Paul C.: The life cycle of the family. *Journal of Marriage and Family Living, 18:*4, 1955; Wells, Robert U.: Demographic change and the life cycle of American families. In Vinovskis, Maris A. (Ed.): *Studies in American Historical Demography.* New York, Academic Press, 1979, p. 529.

46. *Ibid.,* and Glick, Paul C.: Updating the life cycle of the family. *Journal of Marriage and Family, 39(1):*6, 1977.

47. Friedmann, Eugene A.: The Impact of Aging on the Social Structure in Tibbitts, Clark (Ed.): *The Handbook of Social Gerontology.* Chicago, U. of Chicago Press, 1960, p. 132.

48. Bengtson, Vern L.: Generation and family effects in value socialization, *American Sociological Review, 40:*368ff, 1975.

49. Deutscher, Irwin: Socialization for postparental life in Arnold M. Rose (Ed.): *Human Behavior and Social Processes.* Boston, Houghton Mifflin, 1962, p. 509.

50. *Ibid.,* 519-520; the "empty nest" appears to have become a "low impact event" according to George, Linda K.: *Role Transition in Later Life.* Monterey, Calif., Brooks/Cole Pub. C., 1980, p. 82; numerous other studies have reported that children leaving home has not necessarily led to unhappiness on the part of mothers: Axelson, Leland J.: Personal adjustment in the postparental period. *Marriage and Family Living, 22:*66-68, Clausen, John A.: The life course of individuals in Riley, Matilda, W., Johnson, Marilyn, and Foner, Anne (Eds.): *Aging and Society,* Vol. 3: *A Sociology of Age Stratification.* New York, Russell Sage Foundation, 457-514; Glenn, Norval: Psychological well-being in the postparental stage: some evidence from national surveys, *Journal of Marriage and the Family, 37:*105-110, 1975; Harkins, Elizabeth B.: Effects of empty nest transition on self-report of psychological and physical well-being, *Journal of Marriage*

and the Family, 40:544-555, 1978.

51. The impact and potentialities of this change are shown by Uhlenberg, Peter: Cohort variation in family life cycle experience of U.S. females, *Journal of Marriage and the Family, 36*:284-291, 1974.

52. Recent data indicates that the average number of years per child between the time of first marriage and the birth of the last child in the United States in 1977 is 3.4 years. For a family of two children there are 7 years of child bearing and for one of three there are 10 years. After 15 years the children are all in school. Glick, Paul C.: Updating the life cycles of the family. *Journal of Marriage and the Family, 39(1)*:5-13, 1977.

53. Mayer, Thomas F.: Middle age and occupational processes: an empirical essay. *Sociological Symposium, 3*:105, 1969.

54. Jacobson, Paul H.: The changing role of mortality in American family life. *Lex et Scienta, 3*:120, 1966.

55. Hess and Markson, *op. cit.,* p. 255; Hess, Beth B. and Waring, Joan M.: Parent and child in later life: rethinking the relationship. In Lerner, Richard M. and Spanier, Graham B. (Eds.): *Child Influences on Marital and Family Interaction: A Life Span Perspective.* New York, Academic Press, 1978, pp. 241-73.

56. *New York Times,* March 17, 1971; mutual support can involve several generations of family members, Hill, Ruben: *Family Development in Three Generations.* Cambridge, Schenkman, 1970.

57. Lopata, Helen Z.: The widowed family member. In Datan, Nancy and Lohmann, Nancy Johnson (Eds.): *Transition of Aging.* New York, Academic Press, 1980, p. 114.

58. The United States and Canada have approximately 7 percent of the world's population and approximately 70 percent of the world's life insurance. (Private communication from Jack Kier, Professor of Insurance, School of Business Administration, Temple University, Philadelphia, Pa.)

59. Stone, Mildred F.: *A Short History of Life Insurance.* Indianapolis, Insurance Research and Review Service, 1942, p. 27.

60. O'Donnell, Terence: *History of Life Insurance in Its Formative Years.* Chicago, American Insurance Digest, 1936, pp. 195-200.

61. Though in 1671, Jan de Wit had developed the ideas that led to estimations of the values of life annuities based on the probabilities of life at given ages, it was several decades later that adequate life tables for insurance were developed. Jack, A. Fingland: *An Introduction to the History of Life Assurance.* London, P.S. King and Son, 1912, pp. 216-17.

62. A necessary prerequisite to the development of life insurance was the invention of methods for calculating accurate premiums based on known mortality schedules.

63. Jacobson, Paul H.: Cohort survival for generations since 1940. *The Millbank Memorial Fund Quarterly, 42*:48, 1964.

64. Goode, William J.: Perspectives on family research and life insurance. *The American Behavioral Scientist, 6*:58, 1963.

65. Mehr, Robert I.: Changing responsibility for personal risks and societal consequences: premature death and old age. *Annals of the American Academy of Political*

and Social Science, 443:2ff, 1979.

66. American Council on Life Insurance, *Life Insurance Fact Book.* Washington, D.C., 1979.

67. Stone, *op. cit.,* p. 88.

Chapter 7

EDUCATION AND LONG LIFE

THE prolongation of life is directly related to the increasing importance of education. It has, in part, made a greater amount of time available for education. Spending ten to twenty years in the dependent status of student would have been impossible 250 years ago, a time when old age began at age fifty and when the majority of each birth cohort was already dead. In commenting on eighteenth century France, Fourastié wrote ". . . one out of two men died before their twentieth year. Admirable conditions to promote an intellectual civilization! In order to be elected to the academy, it was first necessary to triumph over chickenpox."[1] The relatively short life expectancy did not, by itself, prevent the emergence of a longer period of education. It was also a time when the effect of the precariousness of life and the difficulties of allocating great amounts of surplus wealth to education created a life perspective that inhibited the development of preparatory education for most people. There were some, however, like Montaigne and Pascal who engaged in philosophical reflection and serious scholarship. Our present concern is with the general effect of long life on the increases in time devoted to education.

The history of education reveals a steady progression towards the lengthening of formal education and the enrollment of larger proportions of each age-group in the population. In the United States, eight years of school was a common norm; now, twelve to fourteen is considered appropriate. In 1910, 17 percent of American youth aged twenty-five to twenty-nine years had graduated from high school.[2] By 1979, the proportion had almost quintupled (84 percent for age 25-34).[3] The length of the school year has also increased. In 1876, the average number of days attended by each pupil enrolled was eighty; by 1976, the number reached 178.[4]

College enrollments have greatly expanded. In 1973, almost 45 percent of the males between the ages of eighteen and thirty-four were enrolled in the institutions of higher learning in the United States.[5] Graduate training has grown enormously; from 1920 to 1950, the proportion of students from Harvard College who went to graduate school increased from 20 to 75 percent.[6] As of 1976, 87 percent of Harvard's class of 1971 had enrolled in some postgraduate education.

Throughout history, the majority of men and women were engaged in elementary jobs, hunting or fishing, cultivating the soil, handicrafts, and housekeeping. The skills needed to perform these functions could be learned in a relatively short time. During a lifetime of such work, few changes took place until the individual became physically incapacitated from illness, accident, or old age. In contrast, modern society demands the ability to function in a life fraught with a great variety of social, political and economic (work) contingencies. Contemporary education attempts to respond to modern life by developing a learned capacity. The learning process is often slow and frequently demands painstaking attention to details. Much of modern society rests on the professional, technical, and administrative expertise of men and women who have spent a large part of their lives in preparation for work.

The prevalent explanation for the continuous lengthening of education has been the need for learning how to function in urbanized industrial society. Modern education is both a result and a cause of the knowledge explosion that has spawned the technological achievements of the past century. As mentioned in Chapter 2, some of these early and very basic technical changes took place long before the Industrial Revolution. The next upsurge in technological innovation, sometimes called the Age of Science, came in a period when large surpluses of goods created the conditions of life conducive to a new life perspective, partially made possible by the change in the timing of death. Expectations of long life have provided the economic as well as the temporal basis for undertaking extended educational preparation.

Several social scientists, among them Theodore Schultz, nobel laureate in economics, and Samuel Preston, demographer, have estimated that increases in length of life of youth and adults in low income countries has created strong incentives to invest in schooling and on-the-job training.[7] Moreover, the great increase in infant and childhood survival rates has lowered the real cost of early education.[8] That is, the investment in childhood education is not lost through high death rates in childhood and youth. The results of greater longevity are demonstrated by India's investment in education. During the period of 1951 to 1971, total investment in schooling more than doubled.

As increased life expectancy changed the demographic structure of society, the ages of those who manned the educational organizations were also affected. C.P. Snow illustrates this with reference to King's College, Cambridge: "The average age of the fellows in 1937 was over fifty. In 1870 it was twenty-six. In 1800 it was twenty-seven. In 1700 it was twenty-five. For 1600 the figures are uncertain but the average age seems to have been even less."[9] King's College and a great many other educational organizations that have survived from the past have experienced significant changes due to change in the length of life of the administration and academic staff.

Longevity and the Education of the Young

The education of children and youth has been strongly influenced by the prolongation of life. This can be seen in the changing perspective regarding academic evaluations made by schools. The measure of educational potential is an example: intelligence, native ability, I.Q., and other labels designating levels of performance have been affected. Tests of reading skill, proficiency in the use of numbers, and the ability to rapidly perceive relationships between alternatives, regard speed of learning as an indicator of intellectual endowment. During most of human history, when high mortality rates resulted in many premature deaths, speed in learning served as a crucial criteria in the occupational selection process. Unless the child possessed superior capabilities at an early age, he or she had little chance of rising above the traditional unskilled, domestic, or artisan occupations essential to near-subsistence economies. Speed of learning, as a mark of the talented, has a very long history — small wonder that it has survived so well despite recent reservations among some psychologists.

Contemporary concern with education at the lower socio-economic levels of society has led to the realization that rapidity of learning may not be an infallible indicator of basic intellectual potential. The concept of the slow gifted child has been introduced into the social science literature.[10] Reissman notes that the "style of thinking" of culturally disadvantaged children contributes to failure in present-day American schools. He asserts that, although the deprived child thinks more slowly and requires more examples before he gains insight, it does not necessarily imply an inherently low level of intellectual ability. That is, Reissman denies the validity of assuming a relationship between speed of learning and intellectual capacity. Speed in learning may be the result of culture and early training as well as certain genetic factors.

We need not deny that over the course of time, the children born into some social groupings will have a slightly more favorable gene pool than those born into other groups.[11] However, no measures of intellectual capacity can measure inherited characteristics with any degree of accuracy. In addition to this, the standard methods for determining academic potential fail to account for differences in temperament, rate of maturation (physical as well as mental), family and peer group background, and the host of motivational factors that originate and function in the social milieu of classroom and school.

The number of people who exhibit academic potential, but lack the speed of performance required by the usual achievement tests, gives added support to the conception of the slow learner. The premium placed on speed of learning declines the further one proceeds through the educational system. Ultimately the motivation to work hard in school takes precedence over the measures of attainment provided by standardized tests. It is frequently asserted that persistence is the most important prerequisite for attaining the Ph.D. It would appear that the phenomenon of the slow learner as well as the late bloomer (those who remain unmotivated later than usual) are a result of the extension of life in highly productive industrial societies. In earlier times, a slow beginning usually condemned one to the lowest rung in society.

The increased time available for education, training, and selection of a career encourages a growing number of late bloomers. Longevity has expanded the possibilities for individual choice to a degree formerly impossible under conditions of short life expectancy. Late maturation and the ability to take time needed for education without severe penalties is a new feature in the life of modern men and women.

A wide range of possible career choices in addition to the careful planning and training necessary for pursuing a particular career demands much more time for educational activities than is required in most traditional societies. Modern industrial societies depend upon having a large proportion of the population make a variety of choices between alternative occupations and life-styles. In earlier times, there was a narrow range of available career choices, and these were the prerogative of the few who possessed high social status. Formal education played a small role in shaping the life course.

Contemporary social conditions impose conflicting demands upon educators. Modern men and women face the need for specialization at many points along the occupational spectrum, but the successful person requires special training, psychological and philosophical preparation for flexibility, job mobility, and the new role demands imposed by long life. Increased and varied leisure, a heterogeneous social environment, and rapid social change demand new insight and understanding. In his discussion of the future prospects for Americans, Michael writes "Values and behavior that emphasize and comfortably mesh commitment to tasks; flexibility in learning, unlearning and relearning, constructive attitudes towards an effective use of more hours of leisure, and so on, cannot be taught just at the college level or probably as late as high school; and they cannot be taught by teachers who do not share these values. They probably must be learned in childhood and then modified throughout life as an active learning experience."[12]

How we can be efficiently taught to make the most of a life that is as long and varied as the future may bring is the subject of much writing and endless debate. One incongruity is the notion that we can reduce the time normally taken to earn a college degree. There is a belief that the educational system has been inefficient and that by developing innovations, a school is able to speed up the learning process, thus shortening the time needed for education. The prolongation of life, and tremendous expansion in knowledge, would seem to preclude the possibility of shortening education.

The problem is one that may not call for either shortening or lengthening the time required for a baccalaureate degree. Rather, efforts should be made towards improving the timing, or pattern of sequences, in the educational process. It appears that men and women respond differently to various rhythms of activity — social psychological as well as biological. There is some evidence that long continuous periods of learning devoted exclusively to reading, manipulation of highly abstract conceptions, or meticulous research processes violate some of the social and biological rhythms during certain periods in the life course. The sequence of education year after year, from the nursery through graduate school, may in fact, help defeat some of the objectives of education. The lock-step nature of the system of grade levels and the systematic partitioning of the school year are based more on tradition than the results of scientific research on the processes of learning. Our system of mass education has had a profound effect on the definition and structuring of life, some of which has little to do with formal training or education.

The public school became a powerful standardizing experience after the Civil War, reaching its epitome in the 1960s. Since then, its credibility has been questioned and its hegemony challenged by the increase in private education. The standardization imposed on the first sixteen to twenty years of life is the result of a lock-step system of age-grading that defines individuals by chronological age. This feature of public education has been partially responsible for the development of adolescence, a stage that did not exist prior to the mass education of youth.[13] Age-grading in youth and childhood has become an important aspect of the school environment in modern life.

Age-grading simplifies the administration of schools, public agencies, business, and pension funds. It contradicts, however, the kind of heterogeneity that high technology, increased education, mass media, economic affluence, and long life has created in our society. Age-grading, as it has developed over the past forty to fifty years, has influenced education and our response to age and the aged in ways that distort reality. The failure of our high schools, especially in the large cities, is partially a result of the standardization born of age-grading. The implementation of a standardized curriculum, rigid academic requirements, and specific modes of behavior have resulted in making school alien or irrelevant to the everyday lives of many young people. Recently, a variety of special schools, programs, classes, and social organizations have formed to meet this shortcoming.

At the other end of the lifespan, the Social Security system adopted age-grading by mandating retirement at age sixty-five, thereby setting old age at sixty-five. The movement towards early retirement was also set in motion. As this was taking place, the expected length of life increased, and the degree of instability in death rates and the consciousness of the imminence of death reached the lowest levels in history. Thus, the application of age-grading, which seemed to make some sense for children and youth, has resulted in a rigid definition of old age at a time when length of life has substantially increased.

The age-grading system of education also effectively excludes on the basis of age rather than the need or desire to learn. Fortunately, the standardization that is fostered by age-grading has, to some degree, responded to the realities of change and heterogeneity. Adult education is beginning to become a reality, especially in higher education. The affluence of industrial society and a new perspective of life that is partially attributable to long life have begun to expand our view of life and the way it can be scheduled.

The new conditions of long life have affected conceptions about new appropriate uses of time for adults inside and outside of the educational system. The sabbatical or study leave, which has been a common feature of higher education in the United States, is expanding beyond the ivory towers. Businessmen and government bureaucrats have begun to work towards a system of leave-taking from work for reasons similar to those employed by academicians. As men live longer and the onset of old age increases, preventive medicine, diet, and exercise raise the level of physical well-being of the older person, periodic leave of absence from active work will probably become more common. It could become one of the practices used to relieve some of the urgency for early retirement among certain occupational groups. As vacation planning has introduced a new dimension into the future orientation of an increasing number of occupational groups in modern society, so too would the planning for sabbatical leaves.

Recently, the president of the Federal Bureau of Labor in the German Federal Republic suggested that a one or two year vacation be given a number of years before retirement.[14] This would provide an opportunity for rearranging one's life goals and strategies, as well as define the present and future meaning of one's relationships and obligations to other individuals, groups, and institutions. Such an event might lead to a change of occupation in midlife and would probably encourage a longer and more interesting work life. It would also tend to diminish the trend toward early retirement — a trend that is incompatible with an increasing lifespan and higher levels of health and well being in the later years. The leave from work for a short period could aid in promoting the adaptations required in living a successful long life. Such leaves could be instrumental in fostering new formal and informal educational activities.

The need for specialization and adaptability and the cultural trends toward extended childhood and adolescence demands a highly flexible educational system. The ungraded school, the open classroom, the field experience semester, and repeated starting and stopping of one's college education have become increasingly common aspects of educational experience in the United States. They appear to be tangentially related to the change in life perspective that allows more time for academic exploration, social experimentation, and career selection.

Making Choices and Planning the Life Course

With the postponement of death along the life course, the period of youth has been sociologically extended. This has resulted in the "problem of adolescence" and the prolongation of time to prepare for adulthood. The extension of youth has provided future adults with an increased freedom of choice in the conduct of their lives, a freedom that involves both the opportunity and the responsibility for judging, choosing, and planning the future.

As the number of occupations has increased and the inheritance of occupation from father to son has decreased, the period for making one's initial choice of occupation has been prolonged. The period of formal education has been lengthened, and the necessity of making choices from a larger number of alternative occupations has, in part, accounted for the longer period of choice. However, the full impact of the extended length of education and the perception of the numerous available occupations is mostly felt by those who attend college. Working-class young people probably exercise little conscious choice in entering an occupation. Rather, they tend to move into an available unskilled job in a familiar residence area. The increase in length of life seems to require recognition of the efficacy of education and a commitment to gain the type and amount needed to facilitate suitable occupational choices. Education is a key institution in meeting the social needs resulting from longevity. Moreover, effective prolonged education and self-conscious occupational choice appear to be closely related.

The variety of occupations available in the United States are listed in the *Dictionary of Occupational Titles* and number over 30,000. Availability of many alternatives for work creates a need for the time to explore many options. The emergence of new patterns of exploration and choice contributes to a perspective that includes rationality and planning. The period of youth that is devoted to the choice of occupation and life-style has taken on qualitative changes.

Contemplating the nature of life and exploring and making plans for the future based on rational decision making are related to the decline of a fatalistic view of life. It is a view that relies heavily on fate or God's will as explanatory concepts. Kurt Back has considered the relationship between fate and several major demographic factors.[15] He discusses the possibility of controlling "demographic fate," that is controlling such factors as mortality, fertility, migration, marital selection, and occupational choice. He refers to some of the conditions for individual decision making that involve the realization the variables of fate can be controlled. These conditions are (a) "The actor must know that a decision can be made in the situation, and the 'action' must be known to be technically possible and ethically permissible"; (b) "The person must have the motivation and values to make a definite decision; for instance, he must have a certain career orientation, residential preferences, or be convinced of the value of a planned family"; and (c) "He must have the psychological makeup and live in a social environment which makes it possible for him to act on his choice."[16] Back points out that, even in an unfavorable situation, the above conditions may effect decisions that maximize the individual's control over the variables of fate.

The probability of long life promotes a type of social structure that increases the possibility of Back's conditions being present. This contributes to the realization that the variables of fate can be controlled. In effect, freedom from the imminence of premature death promotes an orientation towards life that includes a greater em-

phasis on rationality and concern about the future. This is not meant
to imply that the realization of a long life is the most important fact;
it is merely one of several important factors that provide the basis for
a control of fate.

Increase in length of life and the corresponding need for planning
and preparation will influence the nature and intensity of the efforts
expended. Along the same path of social action and reaction, an increase in effort will, in turn, change the level of planning, training,
and learning demanded throughout the society. The greatest effect
will be seen in those strata of a population that possess the sociocultural orientation and life-styles that contribute to the realization
that long life has important personal consequences. Knowing that a
decision can be made and that not making a decision will have important consequences increases planning and action.

The prerequisites for participating in a technological society,
coupled with long life, make the recent demands for surrendering
the world of affairs to those under thirty incongruous. During the
1960s, hippie life-styles and rhetoric rejected a concern for the
future, hence delaying personal long-term planning. This may have
been a manifestation of a social consciousness that included some
awareness of longevity. The avoidance of planning and rejection of
achievement orientation on the part of the hippies may have resulted
from the knowledge that there was time for testing and experiment-
ing with various life-styles. It is also possible that it was apparent to
them that overt rejection of rational planning and the linear approach to life embodied in the usual bureaucratic careers in business
and government were some of the most effective ways of declaring
one's independence. Ironically, while they insisted on freedom from
parental and institutional controls, they still remained somewhat
dependent on parents, relatives, welfare departments, free medical
clinics, and universities.

The strident demands of that vocal minority of young people
were more like an echo from a world that is fast disappearing than an
indictment of modern society. In the past, it was often only the
youthful who possessed the physical strength and endurance to handle the major tasks of society. In contrast, the demands of modern
industrial society require long and careful education. Under current
educational schedules, the training required cannot be completed
until well into or after the age of greatest physical strength. It has

ability to complete the training programs.

Case studies show that many adults who have been away from formalized school situations for a long time tend to avoid retraining, often fearful that they will not make the grade. "Moreover, the adult who avoids training is likely to have been an early 'casualty' or 'dropout' from the school education system. The less skilled and less literate see no hope of learning new skills by the technique of the once rejected classroom or by methods of training which they associate with the schoolroom situation."[19]

The failure of older workers to participate in training programs is partially the result of prevailing attitudes toward the question of learning ability and age. Not only does the younger person consider the older person seriously diminished in learning capacity, but the middle-aged and elderly believe the same thing. Therefore, the success of training and educational programs is dependent on change in old and deep-seated attitudes.

A focal point of the research that has confirmed the presumption of intellectual decline with age has centered on the intelligence-quotient concept. Despite the history of criticism among educators and others regarding I.Q. research, findings in the past seemed to confirm the notion that ability and intelligence peaks in youth and declines from then on. Recent research, however, involving a reconsideration of the effects of aging on mental and intellectual functions has challenged these findings.

The earlier assumption emerged in 1930. Basing his research on intelligence testing, Louis Terman assumed that I.Q. peaked at age sixteen.[20] Later research involving the Army Alpha intelligence and Wechsler-Bellevue tests revealed the I.Q. peaked in late youth and early adulthood, and then declined. Later on, Wechsler standardized his test for age, and the peak of the I.Q. rose from age twenty-five to thirty-five. In a study by Shaie in 1963, the peak was again extended, this time to age fifty-five.[21] On the basis of subsequent studies Shaie states, "although it is apparent . . . that there is very little age decrement in intelligence, in functions that do not require speeded response or are affected by slowing of reaction time within the individual, there are nevertheless marked differences in performance level between successive generations. For practical purposes this means that although many older people are functioning at least as well as they did when they were young, still the young of today function at a much higher level than those who were young fifty years ago."[22] In effect, the findings of social science now reveal that the problem of age and intellectual ability is one of obsolescence rather than loss of capabilities due to aging.

Unfortunately, the knowledge that aging does not decrease I.Q. will not diminish obsolescence. The process by which homo sapiens are inducted into human society through early and continuous socialization enhances the prospect of obsolescence. Early socialization to contemporary and time-bound attitudes, values, and expectations is continuously reinforced by one's peers, who in turn, are members of one's birth cohort. This learning forms a powerful base affecting personality, intellectual focus, perspective on learning, and the utility and value of varieties of knowledge. Since we tend to keep an eye on members of our own birth cohort throughout our lives, the acceptability and appropriateness of early norms and perspectives become quite pervasive. We gauge our own life progress by comparing ourselves to our peers and others who are members of our cohort. In effect, we, with our age mates, tend to hold on to and perpetuate earlier shared norms, values, and knowledge. Frequently, much of this knowledge is obsolete.

In the past, a person's birth cohort diminished steadily by death during youth and adult life. The rate of loss was variable and unpredictable. This left one with the imminence of one's own demise, and a lack of generational peers with whom to compare oneself. Thus, uncertainty about the future and a loss of the past as embodied in one's peers affected the perspective of those who advanced in age. Under such circumstances, the future orientation and psychological risk-taking required to participate in the educational activities needed to avoid obsolescence might not be forthcoming.

Although early socialization has a powerful influence on everyone, modern society and long life may ultimately result in social and psychological conditions that make obsolescence more open to solution than in the past. The redefinition of old age, the awareness of the possibility of long life through the stability of death rates, and the diminution of the imminence of death may help to promote a life perspective open to new ideas and experiences. Education and retraining could become a central component in this new perspective. This occurrence will require, among other things, the knowledge and attitudes necessary to separate the age changes occurring in one's body from those involving one's mental and intellectual capacities. The latter do not follow the same downward path. This implies a degree of intellectual sophistication that may not be as prevalent as one might wish.

At the present time, the majority of the elderly are poorly educated. The large-scale improvements in literacy and education are of such recent origin that they have not fully influenced the lives of the present-day elderly. This situation is changing quite rapidly. The elderly of today were born between 1900 and 1915. They matured during and after World War I, a time when new strides in expanding education were underway. The rapid increase in educational levels and the accompanying technological and social changes have created a substantial cultural gulf between the current elderly, the middle-aged, and the young. It has had negative consequences, especially for the aged. Glick has observed "Perhaps as the end of the century approaches, when the elderly will differ less in education and social background from the rest of the population, the public will move more in the direction of treating the elderly as 'people' rather than 'old people,' with each being considered on his or her own merits."[23] The flow of younger more educated cohorts into the ranks of the elderly will undoubtedly have an effect. At present, education, which takes place primarily in childhood and youth, despite its attempt at comprehensiveness, does not prevent obsolescence in middle and old age. In addressing this problem Ryder states, "Perhaps the most sensible way to solve the problem (of obsolescence) would be for us to shake off the shibboleth that all education must precede all labor force participation. Why should we not contemplate opening the doors between the world of work and the world of education throughout the entire life span?"[24] Best refers to the time gained since the turn of the century: "In 1900, when the average life expectancy at age twenty was forty-two years, the notion of obtaining all of one's schooling in youth in preparation for adulthood was a sound idea. Today life expectancy at twenty is about fifty-five years, and the idea of recurrent education throughout longer lifespans is both reasonable and increasingly common."[25]

The new developments in the lives of women have had a decided effect on conceptions relating to recurrent or intermittent education. The awareness among many middle-aged women that their life expectancy fully warrants heavy investments of time and money in education is another manifestation of the consequences of long life. The rapid social change in the roles of women and the new norms of aging have begun to promote a positive orientation towards a future that goes beyond middle age. It is here that participation in education has had an important effect in giving flexibility to our ideas of when and how one can become formally educated.

It appears that continuing education and lifelong learning are not simply programs that may give the ambitious added opportunities or provide the retired with an interesting pastime, but may prove socially necessary. This point of view gained national recognition when, in 1976, Senator Walter Mondale authored legislation entitled The Lifetime Learning Act. An Office of Lifetime Learning was established to coordinate the support for adult learning materials, curricula, and facilities.[26] Federal support was also given to the *Elderhostel* program, which was initiated in New Hampshire in 1975. This is a higher education program for persons sixty and over. For a modest price, they can enroll in week-long academic programs during the summer. Elderly students participate in classes and share educational experiences with younger students at over 230 colleges and universities in the United States.[27]

An orientation toward lifelong learning requires an educational atmosphere that emphasizes individualized learning and a strong sense of self-confidence as learner. Current practices still emphasize competitive learning based on failure or success and governed by a socially based system of rewards and punishments. Failure to change our approach makes the prospects for maintaining status and occupation in late middle and early old age poor. If lifelong education were integrated into the social and economic fabric of society, far-reaching consequences might result. Not only would obsolescence decrease, but this development might disengage education from social status to such a degree that having credentials would no longer entitle one to a higher status job.

The assigning of status to those whose education goes beyond that of the average person is a deeply rooted social practice. With the democratization of access to education and the preponderance of average ability as the basic characteristic of the educated population, educational credentials are losing their place as a prime criterion of status. The development of intermittent lifelong education could result in a gain for society. Such an eventuality would impose greater accountability on experts. An increase in the qualitative importance of education and a decrease in the quantitative (years and degrees) and symbolic aspects would improve the effectiveness of our educational institutions.

We have recently come through a time when the family was the basis for one's status and wealth and provided social position and economic opportunities. The old family based system for assigning class and status gave way to the need for educational credentials. A college education has become a necessary criterion for higher status and income in entering the ranks of adulthood and work. The legacy of a thriving business and a respected position in the local community is no longer the key to a place in the rising middle class.

Our present-day status system generally functions to equate educational credentials with social value and expertise, even when the education considered does little to enhance job performance. Despite this fact, formal academic credentials almost automatically mean higher entry level income and larger increases later on. A system of lifelong education would embrace the pragmatic aspects of education and thereby reduce its importance as a criterion of status. Greater emphasis on performance would change the basis for evaluation.

Relating education specifically to performance and reducing its symbolic aspect as a criteria for job entry and status allocation would ultimately force educational institutions to perform in accordance with their promises. This would create accountability. Grades, certificates, and degrees would then become of greater interest to prospective employers than to colleagues, families, and friends.

The early obsolescence of many workers, white- and blue-collar, and the failure of our educational system to provide timely knowledge throughout life are forcing changes in education and its social function. Such changes would do much towards meeting the challenges of long life in a rapidly changing society.

REFERENCES AND NOTES

1. Fourastié, Jean: *The Causes of Wealth.* Translated and edited by Theodore Caplow. Glencoe, Ill., The Free Press, 1960.
2. Wattenberg, Ben J. and Scammon, Richard M.: *The U.S.A.: An Unexpected*

Family Portrait of 194,067,996 Americans Drawn from the Census. New York, Doubleday 1965, p. 212.

3. U.S. Bureau of the Census: *Statistical Abstract of the United States: 1971,* (92nd edition). Washington, D.C., 1980, p. 148.

4. U.S. Bureau of Census: *Abstract of the United States: 1980,* (101st edition). Washington, D.C., 1980, p. 153.

5. U.S. Bureau of Census: *Statistical Abstract of the United States: 1974,* (95th edition). Washington, D.C., 1974, p. 112.

6. Parsons, Talcott: Toward a healthy maturity. *Journal of Health and Human Behavior, 1:*168, 1960.

7. Rati, Ram and Schultz, Theodore W.: Life span, health, savings, and productivity. *Economic Development and Cultural Change, 27(3):*409, 1979; Preston, Samuel: Causes and consequences of mortality declines in less developed countries during the twentieth century, Mimeographed, New York, National Bureau of Ecomonic Research, 1976.

8. Rati and Schultz, *op. cit.*, p. 412.

9. Snow, C.P.: *The Masters.* London, Macmillan, 1951, Appendix, p. 361.

10. Reissman, Frank: *The Culturally Deprived Child.* New York, Harper and Row, 1962, Chapter 7.

11. Jencks, Christopher: Social stratification and higher education. *Harvard Educational Review. 38:*293, 1968; Eklund, Bruce K.: Genetics and sociology: a reconsideration. *American Sociological Review. 32:*173-193, 1967.

12. Michael, Donald N.: *The Next Generation.* New York, Random House, 1965, p. 83.

13. Hirschhorn, Larry: Post-industrial life: a U.S. perspective. *Futures, 11(4):*287-98, 1979.

14. Rosenmayr, Leopold: Achievements, doubts, and prospects of the sociology of aging. *Human Development, 23:*58, 1980.

15. Back, Kurt: Demography — from impersonal fate to inter-personal control. Paper presented at the annual meeting of the American Sociological Association, Chicago, Illinois, 1965.

16. *Ibid.,* p. 8.

17. This expression of a professional norm may not be functional for maximum achievement among professional peers, but rather for maintaining the closure and exclusiveness sought by organized professional groups.

18. U.S. Senate. *Developments in Aging,* 1976. A Report of the Special Committee on Aging. Washington, D.C., U.S. Government Printing Office, 1976, p. 147.

19. Belbin, Eunice and Belbin, R.M.: New careers in middle age. In Neugarten, Bernice L. (Ed.): *Middle Age and Aging: a Reader in Social Psychology.* Chicago, Ill., University of Chicago Press, 1968, p. 343.

20. The summary material of research on age and intelligence presented here is taken from the excellent article by Schaie, K. Warner: Age changes in adult intelligence. In Woodruff, Diana S. and Birren, James E. (Eds.): *Aging: Scientific Projectives and Social Issues.* New York, Van Nostrand, 1975, pp. 111-151.

21. *Ibid.,* p. 118.

22. *Ibid.,* p. 120; Horn, J.L.: Intelligence, why it grows, why it declines. In Hunt,

J.M. (Ed.): *Human Intelligence.* New Brunswick, N.J., Transaction Books, 1972.

23. Glick, Paul C.: The future marital status and living arrangements of the elderly. *The Gerontologist. 19*:309, 1979.
24. Ryder, Norman O.: The future of American fertility. *Social Problems, 26(3)*:366-7, 1979.
25. Best, Fred: *Flexible Life Scheduling.* New York, Preager, 1980, p. 9.
26. U.S. Senate Special Committee on Aging: *Developments in Aging: 1976.* Washington, D.C., U.S. Government Printing Office, 1977, p. 171.
27. U.S. Senate Special Committee on Aging: *Developments in Aging: 1978.* Washington, D.C., U.S. Government Printing Office, 1979, p. 180.

Chapter 8

CLASS, STATUS, AND LONG LIFE

THE increase in duration of life generally benefited all strata of Western society, but the rate of improvement varied considerably from one part of the population to another. Privileged classes began the period with an advantage, and to some degree, maintained it ever since. During wars, plagues, and lesser epidemics, the possibility of escape from the towns to their castles in the country lent some protection from disease and death.

The frequent havoc wrought by plague and famine had important effects on the social structure of society. Sartre wrote

> The Black Death brought an increase in the wages of farm workers in England. Thereby it obtained what only a concerted action on the part of the peasants could otherwise have obtained (and such action was inconceivable during that period). What is the source of this *human* efficacy in pestilence? It is the fact that its place, its scope, its victims, were determined ahead of time by the government; the landowners took shelter in their castles; the crowding together of the common people is the perfect environment for the spreading of the disease. The Black Death acts only as an *exaggeration* of the class relations; it *chooses*. It strikes the wretched, it spares the wealthy.[1]

One may argue about the relative degree of suffering sustained by the various classes from disasters such as the plague. Until the early part of the twentieth century, however, the differences in length of life definitely favored the upper strata. In England in 1901, "people in the upper class would expect to live for nearly sixty years, but those at the very lowest level for only thirty: paupers were still, in fact, as short-lived as the whole population in Stuart times."[2] Roundtree, the great historian and student of English poverty, observed that laborers were underfed throughout most of their lives.[3] Mothers were malnourished while they carried their children, and the children grew up with malnourishment.

Unpredictability regarding illness and death was the lot of

everyone, although there probably have been differences in mortality rates due to status position since the development of agrarian life. The fortuitousness in the timing of death and its high frequency and apparent imminence gave the impression that it ignored social distinctions. For most people 200 years ago, death had little respect for either peasant or nobleman. The statistical differences in mortality were not readily apparent between the upper and lower levels of society.

It was probably not fully evident that there were definite mortality differences between the social strata until the seventeenth and eighteenth century. The discovery by medical men of the awesome rates of death and disease among the poverty-ridden lower classes of London led to early attempts of sanitation, establishment of lying-in hospitals, and foundling homes.

Since the discovery of great differences in mortality that occurred concurrently with urbanization and the development of industrialization, the greatest gains in length of life have accrued to the lower strata.

A recent summary of studies that deal with differential mortality between social strata in a variety of societies indicates that the greatest differences are between the lowest class and all of those above it.[4] Differences between the middle and upper strata have diminished, and, in some instances, have largely disappeared. The conquest of infectious diseases has been critical in narrowing the class differences among all but the lowest levels. Antonovsky's findings indicate that class differences in death rates are consistently the greatest for those in the middle years of the life course. The differences tend to peak at thirty to forty-four years of age and after that decline and tend to disappear after age sixty-five. The data indicates that differences of this nature ultimately represent preventable deaths.

As the average duration of life becomes approximately the same for the majority of a population, the earlier historic status difference begins to lose its importance. Similarity of long life expectancy gives men and women a critical type of equality, although they may be dissimilar in class and status.

Though generally not considered a status factor, increased longevity gives people the opportunity to see their children live to maturity and to plan a future that introduces a necessary factor in realizing social mobility. When most people share similar chances for a relatively long life, the importance of the added time is obscured. However, long life appears to have had a highly significant impact on the status structure of modern societies.

Long Life and Social Mobility

Long life provides one of the important conditions for intergenerational (between generations) social mobility. To conceive of a level of social mobility that could affect the stratification structure of a society, we also must presuppose an average length of life after biological maturity that is long enough to make mobility possible. Through much of human history, men and women usually did not live long enough to be socially mobile. It could be argued that during most of man's presence on earth, societies have lacked either sufficient stratification or had systems so rigid and closed that the question of social mobility was largely irrelevant. Not until developments such as industrialization, population growth, urbanization, increased longevity, and new perspectives of life began to be felt did substantial levels of social mobility become prevalent.

Prior to the modern period of low mortality rates and long life, some did live fairly long lives, but the imminence of death and the social norms defining old age inhibited most people from attempting to change their station in life. Since long life was unusual, those who lived on were defined as old by the age of fifty to fifty-five. Typically, in an historical sense, the social norms of middle and old age did not encourage or even allow behavior that encouraged mobility. In present-day society, it may be argued that whatever social mobility one experiences, has taken place prior to the late forty's or early fifty's. This is especially true for those whose mobility rests upon credentials that are acquired by going to college. For those who move up continuously after entering their primary career, the peak period occurs at the point that was defined in the past as the beginning of old age, forty-five to fifty-five. Among professionals in modern society, these are the prime years of peak performance and productivity, and old age is viewed as twenty to twenty-five years away.

In general, the distribution of power, wealth, and prestige is closely related to age in modern society. Ryder observes that "most adult roles are located in hierarchized structures" and thus tend to be graded along age lines. "In the majority of occupations, a steadily upward progression of status occurs through most of the age span."[5] This generalization, however, applies primarily to those who follow careers. Lower- or working-class work histories do not usually conform to an upward progression; rather, earnings and prestige reach a plateau soon after the young man or woman is initiated into the world of semi- or unskilled work. In fact, a person of twenty often draws a higher wage than the long-term employee of forty-five to fifty, for reasons that are related to physical capability.

The relationship between longevity and perspective of life has been a recurrent theme. Under certain social conditions, long life may encourage long-range planning, saving, and preparation through education and learning, all of which frequently are the prerequisites for mobility in modern society. Though the Protestant Ethic was one of the important ideological components in the development of middle-class mobility-oriented modern societies, it is not directly linked to long life.[6] The potency of the Protestant Ethic is said to originate from the corruption of Calvinistic emphasis on predestination. Since man's fate in the hereafter was predestined, according to the Calvinists, it meant that there was little one could do to improve one's ultimate place in the afterlife. Nonetheless, one was still encouraged to work hard and live by God's law. However, to ordinary men and women, material success in this world came to be viewed as a sign that one was among the elect. This corruption of Calvin's original doctrine had a powerful effect in promoting an ethic of work, saving, planning, and much of the behavior that was highly instrumental in facilitating social and economic mobility. As the ethic of work developed, longer life and less uncertainty relating to death also become features of human life. Though no claim can be made that long life was a causal agent in the emergence of the work ethic, it facilitated a number of the factors that gave impetus to the high value of work.

In contrast to the relationship between longevity and the ethic of work, long life has also influenced human conceptions of leisure. The social expectation for newly retired people is to enjoy some well earned leisure time. This becomes the basis for life after retirement. Furthermore, the affluence of wealth and living time may have helped to spur the contemporary rejection of many aspects of work. A conception of life that gives leisure a priority over many work activities, formerly believed to be morally necessary, is beginning to replace the work ethic.

From the viewpoint of the student of stratification, many former-ly class-limited leisure pursuits have become democratized. Social mobility and affluence have been key factors in fostering this change in the scope of leisure activities. In effect, a much larger proportion of the world population has not only developed perspectives of life that include rational planning for family size, mobility, and retire-ment, but has developed life-styles that make leisure and play im-portant elements. Among the middle classes, the style of leisure that is viewed as important in this context involves active participation, but is not defined as work. It includes activities such as sports away from home (skiing, canoeing, backpacking, and camping). They usually demand advanced planning and stability and freedom from the imminence of tragedy and uncertainty that characterized life prior to the control of premature death.

Age and social mobility are related to the status of one's residen-tial area in the United States; research indicates that there is a "tendency toward upward social mobility by residential area as age increases. . ."[7] This is found to be true for both higher and lower socioeconomic areas of the city. That is, by living long enough, a family will generally improve its residential status over time. Short life and its accompanying uncertainty serves as a block to this type of mobility, particularly at the lower status levels. Since few studies give the variable of age an important place in the design, relatively little is directly known about residential mobility and long life.

Geographic mobility is a social phenomenon that is related to social mobility, and is frequently mentioned in the same context. Travel for enjoyment and changing one's residence from one geographic area to another are affected by the increased duration of life. In a world of imminent death, moving away from one's home community or planning for a future were either unthinkable or morally suspect. As a result, voluntary geographic mobility was very low. Since some kinds of social mobility are contingent upon geographic mobility, the inhibition of the latter would have conse-quences for social mobility.

At the level of group mobility (differing from individual mobility), long life has meant that age cohorts maturing in the population of modern societies have experienced a wide range of social and cultural changes during their lifetimes. "In some instances, these changes have distributed income and status advantages to segments (cohorts) of the population who began their working lives with few prospects for real gains in these areas."[8] This becomes evident when considering the history of most professional occupations. Whether or not these changes will continue to take place in the stratification of modern society is a matter of conjecture.

Shifting the focus from *intergenerational* mobility to *intragenerational* (mobility within a person's own lifetime), we find that the change in the timing of death and the consequences of longevity have had a direct effect.[9] Extended life allows more time for education prior to entering one's chosen vocation. A comprehensive modern educational system enhances the potentialities for intragenerational mobility. A longer active life can mean that first, second, and even third jobs are not as crucial in detemining one's ultimate occupational commitment as they are under conditions of shorter life. In some occupations, intragenerational mobility occurs later than in others. Long life allows for a variety of different time sequences in mobility.

Intragenerational social mobility is a more immediate or commonplace phenomenon than intergenerational mobility. Longevity has given impetus to this type of mobility, however, since intragenerational mobility does not necessarily imply a rise or fall in income. Though status and prestige may change, one cannot argue that the increase in this type of mobility has had serious effects on the distribution of wealth during a given time period. Nevertheless, the distribution of income for the individual or family throughout the lifespan has been affected by longevity, and this, in turn, is having profound effects on the structure of modern society. Longevity has changed the income curve for individuals and families. The curve rises in early adulthood and middle age. It may be gradual or sharp up to a certain point, and then tends to level off. At the latter stage, the added increments, if there are any, are probably equal to, or only slightly above, increases in the cost of living. The curve usually declines with old age and retirement.[10] It is the last segment of this curve that is the result of longevity. Some of the impact of this phenomenon can be seen; a large percentage of those living in poverty are the ones who have survived long enough to feel the effects of declining income. This is not meant to suggest that the aged were not poor in agrarian or other types of preindustrial society. The primary consideration here rests on the number of people that presently survive to advanced old age.

There are few studies available that spell out the relationships discussed here. Other related social knowledge implies that a set of new dimensions, including those mentioned, have emerged and must be dealt with in attempting to relate longevity and social mobility.[11]

Age, Consumption, and the Use of Status Symbols

One of the most discernible features of any stratification system is seen in the acquisition and display of status symbols. The consumption of material goods may have social significance in ways other than relating to status and prestige, but for present purposes this aspect is most relevant.

Material goods have one or more social functions: utilitarian, aesthetic, or symbolic.[12] To some people, a Rolls Royce or a beautiful piece of antique furniture may fulfill all three functions, whereas an original oil painting or a diamond ring will only have the latter two functions, and a diploma would only possess the third function. Few consumer goods, with the exception of certain staple foods and personal objects such as toothbrushes, arch supports, and so on, are exempt from having some kind of *symbolic function*.

The high level of affluence, a vast array of consumer goods, and diversity of occupational and status communities in modern society has helped create a large number of status indicators. Age or position in the life course has an influence on the acquisition and use of status symbols. With long life becoming commonplace rather than exceptional, a new dimension has been added to the analysis of status and life-style. Our status concerns change as we pass through the life course. This has consequences for consumption patterns and the acquistion and use of status symbols.

At least five of the broad ages of life currently used in social science literature involve individual and social changes that alter previous patterns of consumption. The five ages when status consumption occurs are (1) adolescence, (2) young adulthood, (3) middle age, (4) late maturity, and (5) old age. Age and position in the life course must be considered in an analysis of status-oriented consumption.

Despite the fact that many social commentators and social scientists have observed that modern industrial society is essentially consumption oriented, very few scientific studies have attempted to analyze this change. Most of the marketing studies have tended to ignore the elderly consumer.[13] This orientation has, however, recently begun to change. Consequently, questions abound as to the differences in consumption patterns. There appear to be certain goods and services that are generally consumed more frequently by persons middle-aged and older. For example, they appear to be the major consumers of the best and most varied food and drink. They also comprise a proportion of those who do most of the transcontinental and off-season intercontinental traveling.[14] They may also be the prime culture consumers.[15]

Economic factors impinge on many of the symbolic aspects of life-style. Individuals in the middle strata of society tend to reach their peak in occupational rank, achievement, and income during the age decade between forty-five and fifty-five. That is, they are able to pay for theatre and concert tickets, European tours, paintings, meals in more expensive restaurants, larger automobiles, and more frequent services from hairdressers, cleaning women, or psychiatrists.[16] In some instances, one or more of such items may become symbols of status for the various status communities (individuals and groups sharing a similar life-style, which is based on more than income or occupation) that comprise the middle levels of modern society.[17] Thus, the prevalence and utility of status symbols for the middle levels will vary both by age and status community.

Students of social stratification have often emphasized the importance of the home as a status symbol. It is one of the most costly items of consumption, as well as the locus of a significant part of the life of its inhabitants. Its status value varies with the age of the occupants. A newly married middle income level couple looking for an apartment in the city may find a small one in a run down area that they deem quite satisfactory, but a fifty-year-old couple might find it completely unsatisfactory. The middle-aged couple would be much more conscious of the importance of their home as a symbol of their membership in a status community, a community that has definite norms regarding the proper home. They would also be aware that others at their age level would tend to draw conclusions about their prestige and economic and political influence from the type, location, and furnishings of their home. The young adult couple, not fully identified as to their status community, would generally be less concerned with such matters. This is not meant to imply that young adults are not conscious of the acquisition and use of status symbols, but that the symbolic value of certain objects are different.

The subject of status symbols and life-style cannot be discussed without some consideration of the phenomenon of status striving. Thousands of words have been written regarding the prevalence of status striving among the people of modern industrial society. It has been characterized as reaching panic proportions.

Despite the inferences drawn from Mills and Packard,[18] all middle level people are not panic stricken by the possibility of falling behind in a race involving status striving. Impressionistic evidence indicates that while some groups or status communities may evidence status behaviors that exhibit panic many others do not.

Increased affluence and the wide variety of consumer goods in modern societies provide a wide choice in the acquisition of status symbols. The symbolic value of many material objects has become confused and obscure. With a large portion of the population able to choose and buy many potential status symbols, there ceases to be common agreement on the status value of most material objects. Objects that may have high value for one status has none in another. Furthermore, once the symbol is acquired, the status audience viewing it may be relatively small and specialized.

Affluence, technology, division of labor, and subsequent democratization of many symbols have contributed to the demise of the most universally esteemed status symbols. Now, only one's peers, members of one's own status community or occupational grouping, know the symbolic value of one's latest acquisitions. It does not mean that status symbols are dissappearing, but that their critical importance in social relations is declining, due to blurred value. Long life has contributed to the change in the importance and meaning of many status symbols.

The democratization of status symbols is closely related to the democratization of leisure. It was one of the early major symbols of status.[19] As time passed, certain leisure activities, particularly in the realm of sports and personal combat, took on high status value. In recent times, such sports as skiing, golfing, sport fishing, and small boat sailing are enjoyed by broad segments of middle status people.

As a result, they have lost their luster as primarily upper status activities. Traveling by packaged tours or in trailers or mobile homes increasingly involves people in the older age categories, as well as those in middle level status communities.

Longevity has stimulated some interesting speculation on the part of gerontologists. Research on retired persons and some of the communities in which they have congregated reveals pertinent findings in regard to leisure. An increasing number of persons retiring before sixty-five and in good health have had considerably more experience with mobility and leisure activities than did previous cohorts of older persons: ". . . some of those persons will be 'pioneers' in creating new and different life-patterns in retirement."[20] The nature of life prior to retirement influences the acceptability of certain modes of life during retirement. It was found, for example, that retirees who adopt a leisure-oriented life-style during retirement find the planned retirement communities contribute to such a way of life.[21]

From various research findings, Wood infers that

> the development of more flexible life-style in which there is a more even distribution of education, work, and free time throughout the life cycle . . . would have important implications for age norms. If education were not limited to the earlier part of the life-cycle; if an uninterrupted stretch of work from young adulthood to old age were not the standard pattern; if quantities of free time were available to individuals before retirement; if, in sum, individuals were to combine education, work, and free time in an infinite variety of patterns, then age would seemingly become less salient as a determinant of appropriate behavior.[22]

If people develop life perspectives and styles embodying flexibility of the kind envisioned by Wood, many of the present conceptions relating to status and privilege will need revision. A life-style that places education and leisure on a more equal basis with work could mean the end of the work ethic. This would be especially true for those who make much of the importance of work and view leisure as simply recreation that is done in order to pursue further work more effectively. Such a change would mean the eventual decline in the importance of two of the oldest and most potent symbols of status, leisure and advanced education.

With the fragmentation of the stratification structure of modern industrial society, the influence and importance of class norms has declined. When the middle level of society can be characterized as a mosaic of a large number of status communities rather than as a unitary class, the availability and acceptability of pursuing alternative life-styles is greatly enhanced. In turn, the status value outside of one's own status community of any particular status symbol is ambiguous or unknown. Moreover, declines in the value of status symbols combined with the uncertainty regarding their importance would tend to discourage large expenditures of time and money on their acquisition.

Though relatively little is known about the causes of status striving, the resultant behavior is most prevalent from young adulthood through middle age. The later stages of life seem to exhibit a decline in status striving. The major status concerns are with the maintenance of previous gains or maintaining stability at a lower level of consumption and participation during middle age and after. As large numbers of the population move into the age levels that perceive status striving as fruitless or precarious, there is a possibility that attitudes and values of this kind will mitigate against some of the negative aspects of status striving depicted by Mills and Packard.

Though the prolongation of life is only one of the ingredients that may be contributing to a potential decline in status striving, it may ultimately be of greater importance than it initially appears. Not only does longer life add to the concern about the use of leisure time, but as discussed previously in "Longevity and Life Perspective," it also tends to foster a new life perspective. This perspective includes greater attempts to plan ahead and greater willingness to invest more time in preparation for worthwhile tasks and in learning to live in a manner that is more conducive to remaining alive and well even longer. Current attention to exercise and diet among middle-strata Americans are indicative of the latter point.

This predisposition to plan for a longer life does not mean that the confidence and sense of rightness and destiny are shared by the contemporary middle strata. David Reisman has written that a change has occurred among those who would seem most likely to have inherited the legacy of the older middle-class morality, one that embodied the view of a futuristic approach to life. "Many members of the upper-middle class have today lost that feeling of confidence. Their adaptability, their gift for holding and changing opinions, no longer give them the sense that, as individuals and as members of a rising group, they can shape their own and their countries' destiny over time."[23]

It is apparent that the individual futures of men and women experiencing the increased prolongation of life introduces a new factor into middle-strata life-styles. Under contemporary conditions of rapid social change, the awareness of long life is coupled with experience and knowledge that predispose the middle levels to view occupation, class, and family position as relatively precarious or unstable. The awareness of vast change experienced during one's own lifetime and its actual or potential problems and dislocations pose both threats and challenges. Much of the concern of those who are in the transitional period from relatively short to long life is a result of the tensions posed by the quiet revolution in the chronology of life and death.

Long Life, Poverty, and Inheritances

Other factors related to longevity have had an effect on the wealth and services available to the entire population. With trends towards a greater number of people retiring from gainful work, the ratio of dependent people to productive working people increases. Basic requirements such as food, shelter, and clothing must be created by a proportionately smaller population than was true in the past. The aged, out of the work force because they are retired, are joined by children, teenagers, mothers or infants, and the chronically ill and infirm. Together they constitute a very large dependent population. Long life has meant extra years of retirement for the elderly and has increased the ranks of the poor.

A study done in Philadelphia clearly illustrates a relationship between age and poverty:

> Among the segment of the white working class . . . which we sampled, only about 15 percent of those forty-five and fifty-four are poor. The proportion in poverty rises in the fifty-five to sixty-four category, where slightly over a quarter of the respondents are poor. But in the oldest category, those between sixty-five and seventy-nine, the proportion who are poor is twice that of those just under sixty-five. Over half, 55 percent, of the aged are poor. This distribution conforms in general to what we know about the relationship of poverty to age among whites in the urban working class throughout the country.[24]

Long life not only contributes to the ranks of poverty in the

United States, but in general, has consequences for the size of legacies. Since each parental generation will, on the average, live to see its children become middle-aged, the likelihood that the middle-class families will provide their children with much inheritance diminishes. When the parents do die and leave an inheritance, their offspring may be at the peak of their own earning capacity. Such a legacy is of relatively less importance in providing the new opportunities that might have opened had the parental generation died when the children were in their late twenties or early thirties. Also, the parental generation may have spent a much larger portion of the potential inheritance than would formerly have been the case. The high cost of professional care for a proportion of the old-old (over 75) and the extreme elderly (over 85) rapidly depletes the resources of long-lived elderly. The new norms relating to travel and recreation among healthy retired people in the middle class tend to maintain the consumption patterns practiced before retirement. Nevertheless, in most cases, consumption must be somewhat curtailed due to diminished income.[25] The net results of long life, contemporary middle-class life-styles, and expensive maintenance and health care are that inheritances may be proportionately smaller and may become available in a period of lesser need. The most needed legacies that come to young adults may come from grandparents instead of parents.

This development may have the ultimate effect of eliminating the concern over economic inheritance, especially among the middle and lower classes. Therefore, longevity among the middle strata would help maintain the rationalistic and bureaucratic tendencies toward meritocracy. Among the middle classes, extra money is used to provide children with costly, educational experiences and opportunities. Frequently, the economic sacrifices of parents in providing education is charged against what might have been a larger inheritance.

Long life also may have stimulated the formation of new patterns of parental help in such areas as home financing, funds for advanced education, and extra recreational activities. The more affluent parents in the middle and upper middle strata frequently provide a substantial down payment for the purchase of a home for their offspring. Though borrowing money for the initial down payment of a house is illegal, in most places, the funds provided by parents or in-laws are classed as gifts.

Early marriage, coupled with a long and expensive education, has also brought about family-help patterns that involve parental contributions to help pay tuition and living expenses at college. This frequently happens long before the death of the parents.

Longevity and Power Elites

Longevity and the timing of death have important effects on the composition of the groups that wield power in society. Variation in the length of life has important consequences in determining the length of time during which power positions can be achieved, who will control the entry into elite groups, and how long the same individuals will exercise control. The social homogeneity of decision makers, due to slow depletion of a given birth cohort of elite members, is also important.

Longevity and a life perspective conducive to a certain degree of planning and rationality extend the period of life during which an ambitious man or woman choose to work toward the acquistion of elite status. Long life provides an important perception of stability in planning one's future. However, long life also results in counter-forces of instability due to the awareness of rapid social change. Nevertheless, the stability that long life offers can be illustrated by contrasting contemporary life with life in the past. In the past, premature death from flu, small pox, pneumonia, tuberculosis, and typhoid would have periodically killed the head of a business firm, an army general, a king or archbishop, large numbers of specialized artisans, as well as many of one's family and friends. The laborers that were needed to keep farm, vineyard, factory or government operational sometimes died en masse in a brief period of time during plagues or epidemics. It seems plausible that the precariousness of life may have helped foster a tacit acceptance of the rigid stratification structure of feudalism and the strong class norms separating the earlier upper and middle classes from the lower working classes.[26]

Prior to contemporary control over disease and imminent death, efforts to climb the ladder of success could be wiped out by deaths of key individuals. A business venture or an advantageous appointment frequently ended following the sudden death of one or more crucial individuals.

Although the sudden death of key people in the decision-making hierarchies of business and government is serious, even now, large bureaucratic structures develop strategies to minimize the effect of premature or sudden death. This is due to the rational division of labor and relative precision in allocating duties and responsibilities in the decision-making process. Thus, a replacement is much more readily found and trained to take over the vacant position.

Bureaucratic organizations have institutionalized retirement. This has served to speed the rise of younger men to the higher ranks of executive power. In the top echelons, however, the retired sixty-five year-old corporation president frequently gains an influential seat on the board of directors.

In the case of national political leaders, U.S. senators and representatives continue to run for reelection and quite frequently remain active until their eighties and nineties. The charge that we are controlled by a gerontocracy is most relevant when applied to the political sector.[27] The world of business of finance, however, exhibits a number of gerontocracies, although they tend to be shielded from public scrutiny.

Since esteem and success are currently measured in terms of effective power in the economic or political arena, tendencies toward gerontocracy make it difficult for the young adult to gain high position in the established sectors of society. Longevity makes the combination of youthfulness and power more and more unusual except in the new and developing areas of economic and political life. Long life has resulted in a number of large cohorts, a proportion of which have succeeded to positions of power in the recent past, and are remaining in power into old age. The postponement of death and the slower depletion of cohorts that are now in late middle and early old age have left a large number alive and in positions of influence and power. The size of these groups tend to block the rise of many young men.

The rhetoric of the student radicals in the late 1960s frequently alluded to negative aspects of older age-groups by the use of such slogans as "don't trust anyone over thirty." This was stimulated by the apparent gerontocracy in positions of political power, which was partially the result of longevity and the vagaries of electoral politics. The youth revolt and the generation gap can be directly connected to the increased longevity of a group of earlier cohorts that had gained positions of power. These cohorts were being depleted by death or incapacitation at a much slower rate than in the past. Since they had matured and been educated in a period vastly different from that of the young, a generation gap became clearly discernible.[28]

These cohorts were socialized during a time when advanced education was attained by relatively few. Consequently, their attitudes and perspective of life were shaped by a very different social world. Long retention of power by members of these cohorts has helped stimulate the critical stance of youth toward the so-called establishment.

Though longevity is only one contributing factor, it seems that the historical possibility of another Alexander the Great, or similar youthful giant, is now all but impossible. Heroes like the astronauts and cosmonauts tend to be in their late thirties or forties before they are able to fulfill their major functions. Soon the majority of all school teachers, from kindergarten to university, will exhibit a rising median age. Therefore, these important socializing agents, manning one of the largest and most influential institutional structures in modern history, will cease to be influenced by the continued influx of very large numbers of young teachers and administrators.

Rapid expansion in personnel within any social structure and during any short period leads to an elderly population within a couple of decades unless there is a high amount of turnover through death or social mobility. Under stable conditions, death and retirement are the major mechanisms facilitating entrance of the younger cohorts, pariculary when the age structure of the organization in question exhibits a wide distribution of all age levels. Wide age distributions in specific organizations are, for the most part, fortuitous in that little formal attention is paid to maintaining an age range in the various organized units of society.

For a number of years, the younger, more liberal members of the United States Senate have fought to curb the power of an entrenched gerontocracy, with some recent success. Norms regarding the appropriate ages for retirement are currently in flux, even among such exclusive elites as the United States Senate and the Supreme Court.

Resignation from active involvment in positions of power could become institutionalized, though in many instances the present chronological ages of sixty and sixty-five may prove to be too early. With long life, the acting out of a "thirst for power" or "power as a basic force in man" may become considerably modified and cease to be viewed as basic assumptions. Under contemporary conditions of longevity, a large proportion of men and women from the same age cohort can now hold power for long periods of time.[29] If the negative consequences that are attributed to some of the present-day geron-tocracies is well founded, a time may come when enforced retire-ment from power will become institutionalized, though retirement age for most others is becoming more flexible. The social and psychological as well as political and economic effects of a limited tenure in a position of power could have major social consequences.

Long life may encourage the development of a new dimension in life perspective in relation to power-wielding. In the past, voluntary retirement from power seemed incomprehensible. In recent times, college presidents like Goheen of Princeton University and Meyer-son of the University of Pennsylvania have retired early from posi-tions of power and prestige. The length of tenure in top ad-ministrative positions within organizations like universities is cur-rently being discussed. President Meyerson ruled that no ad-ministrator above a certain level will be allowed to serve in the same capacity for more than twelve years.[30] President Goheen had set a maximum of fifteen years on his own term of office. A number of United States senators and congressmen have recently left the con-gress through resignation and early retirement.

Before limited tenure in positions of power becomes accepted, and thus institutionalized, men must come to view life as a con-tinuous whole that constitutes more than one dominant set of social roles such as work, education, and leisure. Other roles, however, will probably have to improve in desirabilty and value before the major occupational roles lose their dominance; especially since those roles provide the avenues to power.

During the past few years, social commentators have observed that a disproportionate number of elderly widows have inherited potentially great fiscal and economic power. Fears have been ex-pressed that these presumably conservative women would have a constraining effect on economic growth by avoiding ventures involv-ing risk. Assertions such as these, though based on certain demographic facts, are generally ill-founded. It is unknown whether rich elderly widows are more conservative than their husbands were. In addition to that, since business and finance usually have not been a normal part of most women's roles, they rarely assume active control over the fortunes left by their husbands. Generally, these widows turn their fiscal affairs over to someone else, usually a male, either a lawyer or financial counselor. He alone, or with the aid of a trust department of a bank, takes over the effective control of the widow's wealth.

In a sense, the disproportionate life expectancy of females over males may have other important, though obscure, effects on the structure of power in modern society. A considerable number of the financial experts who are hired to control the fortunes of rich widows exercise their control within a super institutionalized and insulated legal framework. They may be called the holders of what has been named *faceless power*.

Richard Sennett, who has written of the antidemocratic decision-making process in the highly rationalized structures of modern society, states that ". . . impersonal bureaucracy and faceless power has become the great weapon of the middle classes today over those who do routine labor."[31] A substantial number of fortunes controlled by the faceless representatives of wealthy widows adds to this form of power wielding — a power that may be susceptible to a drift toward irresponsibility or ruthlessness.

Turning from this area to the problems of failure and long life, one sees opposing possibilities. In one way, longevity makes the influence of the personnel dossier and record of transgression over a long life seem particularly inhumane. All past mistakes do not necessarily inhibit the capacity for change. Forgiveness for past mistakes or indiscretions may have to be incorporated into the legal and social norms of the future.[32] Condemning men to decades of punishment for early misdeeds may become an issue in public policy making.

Long Life and the Status of the Elderly

It has often been assumed by many who write about the elderly that modern industrial society has brought a decline in the status position of the aged. There is no doubt that the change from a traditional, agricultural society to an industrial-urban society has imposed many changes in social relations and social organization. There is, however, disagreement among scholars as to whether or not the aged have lost status in the process of modernization.

Much of the controversy rests on the changes resulting from the rise in urbanization and industrialization. "The basis of social status changed dramatically during industrialization from a system based on control of property (land) to one based on control of the means of economic production (factories and machines). The nature of the division of labor also changed with the Industrial Revolution from one based on ascription to one based on achievement. Social status and one's social 'worth' in modern society reflect the premium placed on efficiency, rationality, and productivity."[44]

For some social scientists, evidence indicates that status and power go hand in hand. Diminished power in the economic and occupational spheres of life result in a status loss for the elderly. Dowd defines status as "relative income, health, weeks worked, and education."[34]

Cowgill and Holmes did a comprehensive cross-cultural study of the effects of modernization on aging and point to aspects such as urbanization, technology, and literacy as key elements.[35] They argue that these changes increase the status of the young resulting in a loss for the elderly; for example, education is geared for the younger age-groups. The importance of education is related to science and technology, which have diminished the importance of the elderly. The memory and wisdom of the elders have been replaced by libraries and experts. The conclusions presented by Cowgill and Holmes, however, leave room for considerable variation on the question of status of the aged. They state that for the United States, the conclusion may rest on the definition of status, but on the other hand ". . . that the aged, at best, occupy an ambiguous status. . . ."[36]

Lipman, as have other scholars, has written specifically about "the prestige of the aged."[37] This is a different concept from those used by Dowd, Cowgill, and Holmes. While Lipman's concept involves primarily honor and deference, the latter use concepts including economic level and occupation. Lipman reports that the rural aged of Portugal receive high levels of *ritual deference*. They are treated "as if they were wise and respected," but that behavior often serves as merely lip service to the myths and norms governing treatment of the aged.[38] The result is relatively low status while receiving a superficial ritualistic kind of deference. Other scholars have also questioned the idea that the aged have lost status as a result of modernization.[39]

As already mentioned, the problem may rest on the variability in the definitions of status. If economic position (class) and honor and deference (status) are put together and called *status*, the conclusions drawn from the analysis will be affected. An anaylsis that distinguishes between Weber's concepts of class and status will lead to substantially different conclusions.[40] If status is analyzed as distinct from economic position (class), the difference between the findings of Dowd and Lipman are readily explainable.

A review of the literature on the status of the aged throughout history provides inconclusive results; this is partially due to a lack of uniformity in the definition of status. Dowd concludes that in terms of relative economic power, health, weeks worked, and education the status of the aged has declined with modernization.[41] His definition combines Weber's concepts of class and status. Lipman, Laslett, Neugarten, and Hagestad disagree with Dowd, primarily because their analyses are based on prestige and deference. Their conclusions rest on the use of Weber's concept of status, rather than a composite conception including the two elements of class and status.[42]

When analyses of the status position of the aged is based primarily on income (class), the data fall into a curvilinear pattern. Since income is so readily quantified (dollars, marks, or yen), the concept of status also takes on a predominantly quantitative aspect. As a result, a variety of quantitative factors relating to prestige, honor, and deference are discounted or omitted.

Age is generally ignored in evaluating the importance of various status indicators. It is assumed that the values assigned to some status symbols are uniform throughout the life course. For example, it is tacitly assumed that age need not be considered in the way a person values ownership of property, a comfortable well-appointed home, fashionable clothes, and high income. Youth, young adults, the middle aged, the young old, and the old-old all vary considerably in the precise value that they place on the symbols and objects of status.

Status as a social variable is presumed to behave like income, even though it is not quantifiable in the same way as income and wealth. It is thought to form the same kind of curve over time, rising in youth and falling in middle and old age. It is this decline in status that is the basis for concern. If status is defined as a virtual correlate of income, then aging will necessarily entail a serious loss. Status, however, is properly defined in terms of a particular process of evaluation relating to social definitions that are based on social structure and cultural heritage. Status usually connotes prestige, deference, and honor resulting in a particular life-style.[43] All of these are the result of *social relationships*, which in turn, change continuously throughout the life course.

Some of the social changes are the result of a crisis that frequently signals a change in the life course itself. A number of these crises generally occur toward the latter half of life: children leaving home, retirement from paid employment, death of a spouse, and physical disability are common. Numerous other crises occur in childhood, youth, and middle age, but it is assumed that the earlier crises have less permanent results, and that any losses suffered can be recouped in the future. Whether or not this is true is open to question. Social scientists have yet to develop adequate theories of human development and behavior that allow one to judge the importance of one life crisis against another.[44] The presumption that the crises of the elderly are more serious than those occurring earlier in the life is probably due to the fact that they occur closer to the expected end of life. Many societies also value the activities of the young and physically able more than those of the aged, a value that has been highly functional for most societies throughout human history. It is only in recent times that surplus wealth and longevity have given human life a new set of dimensions that denote a change in the concept of life itself. One of these involves the specific conception of how life can or ought to be lived in late maturity and old age.

The definition of aging has suffered from the same kind of static and organic presuppositions that give the concept of status its simplified quantitative character. It has resulted in the grouping of all elderly people into one category of aged or old. This has contributed to stereotyping, which has placed social restraints on options open to the elderly. Much of the social scientific data indicate, however, that there is great variation as to the exactly when and how these changes occur. Age, like status, must be defined in terms of social relationships, hence as a dynamic conception.

It is becoming evident that scientists are beginning to exercise greater care in the definition of aging. Nevertheless, the semantic legacy regarding old age continues to have a powerful influence on the way we define the last period of the life course.

The great increase in the proportion and number of aged in modern society has increased their social visibility, particularly those who are dependent, ill, or destitute. By inadvertently imposing themselves upon the sensibilities of a large portion of society, they highlight the negative aspects of aging. A contemporary writer refers to the existence of an "elderly mystique" as a self-derogating, hopeless, and socially and psychologically limiting perception of old age.[45] This seems to be a continuation of an earlier view. Shakespeare vividly portrays the negative connotation of old age compared to youth:

> Crabbed age and youth cannot live together
> Youth is full of pleasance, age is full of care;
> Youth like summer morn, age like winter weather;
> Youth like summer borne, age like winter bare.
> Youth is full of sport, age's breath is short;
> Youth is nimble, age is lame;
> Youth is hot and bold, age is weak and cold;
> Youth is wild, age is tame.
> Age, I do Abhor thee; youth, I do adore thee.[46]

Ariés points out that prior to the eighteenth century the old were regarded as ridiculous.[47] Many of Shakespeare's lines also reflect this view. Not only was age viewed as a hopeless or ridiculous stage of life, but the negative effects become very apparent earlier than they do today. He wrote —

> When forty winters shall besiege thy brow,
> And dig deep trenches in they beauty's field,
> Thy youth's proud livery, so gazed on now,
> Will be tatter'd weed, of small worth held.[48]

Cross-cultural materials from anthropology relating to the status of the aged reveal considerable variation, a variation that seems to exhibit extremes in defining the status of the aged. Commenting on the work of Simmons, Williams states, "His data indicate that aging tends to be viewed either as a dismal and hopeless problem or as a hopeful challenge, without much room for neutrality of attitude. Hence, changing positions with age tend to be somewhat problematic in all societies."[49]

There is no precise point in time or condition that connotes old age. Our language customs, however, have yet to recognize this, at least in the vernacular. Old age is thought to begin between sixty and seventy and end ten to twenty years later in death, having gone through at least two substages. The first substage is characterized as the aged person with adequate facilities, good health, and high morale, now labelled the "young old." Such a person can readily hold a satisfactory place in the social environment, whether or not he or she depends on certain individual characteristics. Under stable social conditions, this person will be held in esteem by family, friends, and long-time associates. Therefore, his or her status may be satisfactory.

Perception of one's status is an important aspect of personal life. In a study of retired people, it was reported that only 15 percent of them felt that they were treated with less respect as a result of retirement. Education seemed to be related to perception of status. About one third of those with less than high school education felt that retirement led to a loss of status, whereas only 3 percent of the college education percieved a loss.[50] Nevertheless, since status changes with age, it is often considered to have declined.

Longevity has vastly increased the number and proportion of aged who have lost their capacity to function independently. It is not surprising that these people have low status and tend to depress the overall status of the aged, as well as perpetuate a derogatory elderly mystique. Since, however, longevity has increased by the rise in level of living, nutrition, and certain medical advances, the health and well-being of those who live long is probably much greater than in the past. One might infer that the basic reason for the abhorrence and ridicule of old age in Shakespeare and others was due to the generally deplorable state of health and the resultant living conditions of those who attained advanced age — those who lived beyond youth and who had passed through forty winters.

A counter argument can be advanced. Under conditions of primitive, nonscientific medical care, the high death rate would tend to weed out those who are biologically deficient and thus leave a strong and presumably healthier population to live on through later stages in the life course. Living through some diseases may strengthen the coping characteristics of the human organism. There are, however, countless diseases that weaken and contribute to the increased susceptibility of other fatal or debilitating diseases, such as pneumonia and tuberculosis. Childhood diseases, like measles and rheumatic fever, may leave permanent damage and contribute to ill health in adulthood. Adequate historical data on the level of health, durability, or robustness of our forefathers is almost nonexistent; slight available evidence supports the contention that the past exhibited a low average of physical health and well-being for those who lived beyond the fourth decade. If such were the case, negative connotations of old age could still prevail, even though the few who lived on and were healthy may have been granted a degree of deference, based on their uniqueness and good fortune.

It can be argued that one of the indicators of rising status for a social category is the amount of effort that is expended in meeting the peculiar problems of the population in question. Individually, we have probably always shown personal concern for our own future in old age, even though the likelihood of getting very old is questionable. Collective concern and the allocation of time and resources for coping with the problems of the aged are, however, relatively recent phenomena and directly related to the prolongation of life. As previously mentioned, the concern manifested in the special attention paid to childhood as a distinct period in life is of recent origin, and the same is true for those at the other end of the life course.

Bertrand de Jouvenal has made an interesting observation on this issue. He wrote, "I doubt whether devotion to one's own children has ever before in Western society been as widespread and intense as it is today. But beyond that, we are possessed by the excellent feeling that we stand collectively in *loco parentis* to the whole succeeding generation." He claims that however laudable our concern with the young, "our thoughts are so much addressed to those who came after us that we have little attention left for our predecessors."[51] Until recently, this observation was quite correct. Increased longevity, however, has raised the number of aged above the threshold of public awareness.

Although the emergence of social gerontology signifies a concern with the problems of aging, the younger population in modern society continues to claim a high place in the general system of values and a large part of the available resources. A kind of simple pragmatism regarding human resources seems to prevail. Cottrell aptly states that "Public education of the young is justified by the contribution they may yet make. Worry over the young deviant is multiplied by the years of damage he may yet inflict upon society. The dramatization of the young polio or palsy victim is much easier than it is presenting an appealing picture of the problems of the aged."[52]

An aspect of industrialization that favors the older person is the fact that the importance of physical strength has declined as a criterion of employability. Knowledge, experience, and adaptability are steadily becoming more important as qualifications for employment. Age does not preclude the possession of these qualities. Talcott Parsons argued that the experiences of long life impose the necessity of responding to a continuous "process of renunciation and abandonment of lost objects," particularly in the psychological sense.[53] The loss of parents, friends, missed opportunities, and decline in status have to be faced. Parsons writes, "If an individual has been able to handle these object losses and the transition to new object systems successfully, I think we can generalize that he will have profited in maturity and capacity for such things as judgment, compassion, and the like, and will emerge on a higher level of capacity than before."[54] Current evaluations indicate that most individuals are successful along these lines.[55]

Parsons notes that modern technological society demands roles that require a capacity for dealing with high levels of generality, complex individual and institutional relationships, and wide ranges of interest. He states, "that the roles in which our oldest people have most to contribute, if they have survived the strains of the previous phases of their life-cycle successfully, are roles that stand toward the top of this scale of social development. They are the roles in which the broadest problems of adjustment, orientation, and assumption of responsibility should operate. They are roles where judgment and what is often called wisdom should be at a premium, but where the more confining operative responsibilities are less pressing than in, for example, executive roles."[56] Furthermore, "Another positive aspect of the aging person in such roles is his being in a favorable position to take a broad view and to minimize parochial and personal self-interests. He is likely not to be ambitious in a personal sense, simply because by his age he is excluded from the kinds of opportunity that may be open to a younger person."[57]

Parsons is attempting to show that although the elderly have lost their former status as repositories of useful information and no longer have a monopoly of magical and religious lore, they regain some the their lost status by providing complex social and psychological knowledge and judgment. Ultimately, taking part in some of the important aspects of modern society could take the place of work roles that were reserved for the aged in agrarian society.

National income figures indicate that the average retired American must live on approximately one half of the annual income received during the working years. This represents a serious reduction in economic resources. A prominent scholar on the status of the aged has pointed out that even for those old people who may have a high level of economic resources, they possess an important and devalued status characteristic, namely, old age.[58] This means that even large economic resources cannot be fully translated into high status. Being old results in an unfavorable exchange rate and, therefore, even economic resources lose some of their value in the assignment of a status position in the community. In explaining this problem, Blau states, "pronounced differences in social resources between groups give rise to social processes that transform great average differences in resources (status) between groups into categorical status differences rooted in group membership as such, independent of an individual's own resources."[59] The category of old is highly negative in American society and results in agism and all that it implies.

It appears, nevertheless, that long life and the decline of premature death make a change in this relationship possible and that the status of the aged may improve in time. With the emergence of a perspective of life that is not continually affected by the imminence and fear of death the stereotyping of the aged may decline. Long life has created the basis for an ever widening range of differences in the way people age. New avocations and even work careers are being pursued by people normally defined as old. When we add new scenarios for family life involving late childbearing and rearing, long postparental life, middle age and old age divorce and remarriage, we appear to be on the threshold of new ways of conducting our lives in the latter part of the life course. When differentiation among the elderly reaches a high enough level, stereotyping becomes increasingly difficult. Without stereotying, the categorization referred to by Blau becomes impossible, and both agism and racism rest on the possibility of stereotyping the segments of population in question. With a decline in the ability to invoke stereotypes, differences in esteem and prestige may occur among the elderly. New pursuits of the elderly in all spheres of social, political, and economic life may result in such a variety of new sources of power and status that the general designation of old becomes untenable. We may develop an ideology that places a premium on individual differences among the elderly, which is similar to the way we view the developmental prospects of children and youth. This fits admirably with our general emphasis on individuality and achievement. Long healthy life that is lived in the context of a broad and comprehensive view of increased potentialities in the life course makes variation in status attainment more possible than ever before.

We come back to questions of life perspective and human values. A portion of the whole problem regarding the status of the aged is generated by an insistence that status and class position are the prime measures of success in life. Hence, anything such as age and retirement, which denies one the possibility of maintaining an achieved position, leads to the loss of something very precious. This seems to imply the existence of a law of *status maintenance*, which holds that humans can only be satisfied with a rise in status, but never a decline or loss. Such a conception is open to question. There seems to be no room for the concept of stable status or status changes that alter the values attached to former criteria of status. The conception that the status and class position we acquire during middle age becomes the major criteria of success during our entire life is highly dysfunctional for the last years of the life course. There is evidence that such a view can have damaging consequences during the first twenty years of preparation as well. A somewhat related problem is seen in our current conception of achievement.

The emphasis placed on achievement (achievement potential) throughout the life course as the key to successful aging might be functional if the concept of achievement was broadened from its present-day narrow connotations. The continued reiteration of the achievements (or exploits) of a few aging novelists, scientists, engineers, and round-the-world sailors may be interesting, but not useful information to the vast majority of ordinary aging men and women. From a broader perspective, Cain writes

> . . . are not the old man with a storehouse of tales for neighbor or grand-
> child, the grandmother with skills as a seamstress, the older person who
> has persevered in a job and a marriage and in community organizations (a

church, a union, a lodge), and who has mastered a hobby or an avoca-tional skill also fulfilling achievement potentials? Somehow the geron-tologist must encompass these successes in considering models for the morrow. Actually, the ability of a man to accommodate to what the culture may call failure — failure as a parent or spouse, or as a worker, for example — may be a genuine mark of achievement. Transcending the shattered dream of business or professional success, learning to accept what you are able to become, is an accomplishment possibly made more often by the seemingly insignificant many than by the supposedly signifi-cant few. The peculiar fulfillment of achievement potential represented in the failure of the fisherman in *The Old Man and the Sea* (Hemingway, 1952) is a dramatic illustration of a type of success gerontologists may well ex-amine.[60]

If we are to develop an adequate conception of maturity and ag-ing and a set of social roles and definitions appropriate for a large elderly population, we may have to reorder the cultural value we place on social prestige, economic class, and achievement.

REFERENCES AND NOTES

1. Sartre, Jean Paul: *Search for a Method.* New York, Afred Knopf, 1963, fn., pp. 163-164.
2. Laslett, Peter: *The World We Have Lost.* London, Methuen, 1965, p. 207.
3. *Ibid.,* p. 209.
4. Antonovsky, Aaron: Social class, life expectancy and overall mortality. *The Milbank Memorial Fund Quarterly,* 45(2),Part 6I, 66, (1967); Peller, Sigis-mund: Mortality, past and present. *Population Studies 1 (4):*405-456, 1943; Hollingsworth, T.H.: The demography of the British Peerage. *Population Studies,* supplement, *18(2):*52 ff., 1965; Tietz, C.: Life tables for the social classes in England. *Milbank Memorial Fund Quarterly,* 21:182, 1943; Moriyama, I.M. and Guralnick, L.: Occupational and social class differences in mortality. In Milbank Memorial Fund: *Trends and Differentials in Morality,* New York, 1956; Dublin, Louis I., Lotka, A.J. and Spiegel-man, M.: *Length of Life.* New York, Rolnald Press, 1949, p. 213 ff.; Zito, George V.: *Population and its Problems.* New York, Human Sciences, 1979, p. 227 ff.
5. Ryder, Norman: Cohorts and social change. *American Sociological Review,* 30:857, 1965.
6. Weber, Max: *The Protestant Ethic and the Spirit of Capitalism.* Translated by Talcott Parsons, London: Allen and Unwin, 1930.
7. Willie, Charles V.: Age status and residential stratification. *American Sociological Review,* 25:264, 1960.
8. Stub, Holger, R.: Education, the professions, and long life. *The British Journal of Sociology,* 20:188, 1969.

9. The foregoing section was taken from Stub: *Ibid.*
10. Foner, Anne: Age in society: Structure and change. *American Behavioral Scientist,* (November-December, 1975:157); Riley, Matilda W., Riley, John W. Jr., Johnson, Marilyn E.: *Aging and Society: Aging and the Professions.* Vol. I., New York, Russell Sage, 1969 pp. 210-212.
11. Myles, John F.: Income inequality and status maintenance. *Research on Aging, 3* (2):123-141, 1981.
12. Barber, Bernard: *Social Stratification.* New York, Harcourt, Brace and Co., 1957, p. 136.
13. Waddell, Frederick E.: Consumer research and programs for the elderly — the forgotten dimension. *Journal of Consumer Affairs,* 9:164-175, 1975.
14. Waddell, Frederick E. (Ed.): *The Elderly Consumer.* Columbia, Md., The Human Ecology Center, Antioch College, 1976, pp. 287-296.
15. The term has been defined as those who are involved one way or another — from producers to audiences — in "painting, music, drama, sculpture, dance, literature and the art film." Toffler, Alvin: *The Culture Consumers.* Baltimore, Md., Penguin Books, 1965, p. 19.
16. Schutz, Howard G., Baird, Pamela C., and Hawkes, Glenn R.: *Life-styles and Consumer Behavior of Older Americans.* New York, Preager, 1979.
17. That the middle levels of modern society constitute a "mosaic" of status communities rather than simply being a single unitary social class is explored in: Stub, Holger R.: *Status Communities in Modern Society: An Alternative to Class Analysis.* Hinsdale, Ill., The Dryden Press, 1972.
18. Mills, C. Wright: *White Collar.* New York, Oxford University Press, 1951; Packard, Vance: *The Status Seekers.* New York, McKay, 1959.
19. Veblen, Thorstein: *The Theory of the Leisure Class.* New York, The Modern Library, 1934.
20. Wood, Vivian: Age-appropriate behavior for older people. *The Gerontologist, 2:* Part II, 77, 1971.
21. Bultena G., and Wood, V.: The American retirement community: bane or blessing? *Journal of Gerontology,* 24:209-217, 1969, Normative attitudes toward the aged role among migrant and nonmigrant retirees, *Gerontologist,* 9:204-208, 1969, Leisure orientation and recreational activities of retirement community residents. *Journal of Leisure Research,* 2:3-15, 1970.
22. Wood, *op. cit.,* 1971, p. 78; a more recent discussion of this issue is found in: Best, Fred: *Flexible Life Scheduling: Breaking the Education-Work-Retirement Lockstep.* New York, Praeger, 1980.
23. Riesman, David: Styles of response to social change. *Journal of Social Issues,* 17:90, 1961.
24. Rosenberg, George S.: *The Worker Grows Old.* San Francisco, Jossey-Bass, 1970, pp. 9-10.
25. Schutz, Baird, and Hawkes: *op. cit.,* p. 8.
26. Antonovsky, *op. cit.,* p. 66 ff.
27. Riley Matilda W., and Foner, Anne: *Aging and Society: An Inventory of Research Findings.* Vol. II., New York, Russell Sage, 1968, pp. 476-477.

28. The generation gap seems to make sense in a rational way, even though social science research has failed to reveal any great shift in attitudes and values of youth from those of their parents. The highly vocal and visible college minority made the assumption seem true.

29. As director of the Federal Bureau of Investigation, J. Edgar Hoover served in an important power position within the United States government for almost half a century.

30. *Philadephia Magazine*, Volume 63, May, 1972, p. 196.

31. Sennett, Richard: *The Uses of Disorder*. New York, Vintage Books, 1970, p. 195.

32. The rise of massive record keeping through electronic storage and the use of comprehensive methods of concealed and continuous surveillance has brought forth weeks of hearings in the U.S. Congress on the question of the invasion of privacy and the political dangers of detailed lifelong records of men's private lives. The possibility for the periodic erasing of these electronic records was brought out in the testimony offered in 1971.

33. Dowd, James J.: *Stratification Among the Aged*. Monterey, Calif., Brooks/Cole, 1980, p. 66.

34. *Ibid.*, p. 67.

35. Cowgill, Donald O. and Homes, Lowell D.: *Aging and Modernization*. New York, Appleton-Century-Crofts, 1972, pp. 305-323.

36. *Ibid.*, p. 250.

37. Lipman, Aaron: Prestige of the aged in Portugal: Realistic appraisal and ritualistic deference. *International Journal of Aging and Human Development*, *1*:127-136, 1970.

38. *Ibid.*, p. 135.

39. Laslett, P.: Societal development and aging. In Binstock, R. and Shanas, E. (Eds.): *Handbook of Aging and the Social Sciences*. New York: Van Nostrand, 1976; Neugarten, B. and Hagestad, G.O.: Age and the life course. *Ibid.*

40. Gerth, Hans and Mills, C. Wright; *From Max Weber*. New York, Oxford University Press, 1946, pp. 180-196.

41. Dowd, 1980, *op. cit.*, p. 67.

42. Lipman, *op. cit.*, 1970, pp. 127-136; Laslett, *op. cit.*, 1976, p. 97; Neugarten and Hagestad, 1976, *op. cit.*, p. 38.

43. Gerth, and Mills, *op. cit.*, 1946, p. 186 ff.

44. An attempt to evaluate personal crisis has been made by: Holmes, T.H. and Rahe, R.H.: The social readjustment rating scale. *Journal of Psychosomatic Research*, *11*:213-218, 1967.

45. Rosenfelt, Rosalie H.: The elderly mystique. *The Journal of Social Issues*, *21*:37-43, 1965.

46. Shakespeare, William: *The Ages of Man*. An Anthology Selected and Arranged by Georg Rylands, New York, Doubleday, 1941.

47. Aries, Philippe: *Century of Childhood*. Translated by Robert Baldick, New York, Afred A. Knopf, 1962, p. 31.

48. Shakespeare, *op. cit.*

49. Williams, R.H.: Changing status, roles, and relationships. In Tibbitts, *op. cit.*, p. 270; references are to Simmons, Leo: *The Role of the Aged in Primitive Society*.

New Haven, Conn., Yale University Press, 1945; Old age security in other societies. *Geriatrics, 3*:237-44, 1948; Social participation of the aged in different cultures. *Annuals of the American Academy of Political and Social Science, 279*:43-51, 1952; Cowgill, Donald O. and Holmes, Lowell D. (Eds.): *Aging and Modernization.* New York, Appleton-Century-Crofts, 1972; Press, Irwin and McKool Jr., Mike: Social structure and the status of the aged: Toward some valid cross-cultural generalization. *Aging and Human Development, 3(4)*:297-306, 1972; Palmore, Erdman B. and Manton, Kenneth: Modernization and status of the aged: International correlation. *Journal of Gerontology, 29(2)*:205-210, 1974.

50. Strauss, Aldrich, and Lipman, Aavon: Retirement and perceived status loss: an inquiry into some objective and subjective problems produced by aging. In Gubrium, J. (Ed.): *Time, Roles and Self in Old Age.* New York, Human Science Press, 1976, p. 227.

51. de Jouvenal, Bertrand: The future of the aged. *Spectator, 212*:338, 1964.

52. Cottrell, Fred: The technical and societal basis of aging. In Tibbitts, Clark (Ed.): *The Handbook of Social Gerontology.* Chicago, University of Chicago, 1960, p. 110.

53. Parsons, Talcott: Sociocultural pressures and expectations. In Simon, Alexander and Epstein, Leon J.: *Aging in Modern Society.* Washington, D.C., American Psychiatric Association, 1968, p. 39.

54. *Ibid.,* pp. 39-40.

55. Pearlin, Leonard I., The life cycle of life strains. In Blalock, Jr., Herbert M. (Ed.): *Sociological Theory and Research: A Critical Appraisal.* New York: The Free Press, 1980, pp. 349-360.

56. Parsons, *op. cit.,* p. 40.

57. *Ibid.,* p. 41.

58. Dowd, *op. cit.,* p. 70.

59. Blau, Peter M.: *Inequality and Heterogeneity: A Primitive Theory of Social Structure.* New York, Free Press, 1977, p. 151.

60. Cain, Jr., Leonard D.: Aging and the character of our times, *The Gerontologist, 8*:250-251, 1968.

Chapter 9

WORK, RETIREMENT, AND THE
ECONOMICS OF LONGEVITY

I NDUSTRIALIZATION and the accompanying consequences
of long life have affected several aspects of worklife in modern
society. The daily and annual duration of work, age of entry into
paid work, total work life, leisure time, male-female labor force participation, and aging and retirement are some of the important factors of modern work life.

Prior to 1900, the annual duration of work was approximately
3500 to 4000 hours, which is equivalent to approximately seventy to
eighty hours per week.[1] This heavy work schedule had developed in
European agriculture and was initially adopted by industry. In
agriculture, however, the rhythm of work varied. In spring, early
summer, and at harvest time, the work day was long and intense,
while in the winter it was short and leisurely. Whether or not such a
rhythm suits human beings better, as stated by Fourastié, remains a
matter of conjecture.[2] Nevertheless, Fourastié is probably correct in
asserting that a work schedule of seventy to eighty hours per week
could not have been permanently sustained in the large urbanized
industrial centers. It was, however, in force until the twentieth century.

A comparison of the time budgets of adult workers during the
traditional epoch (the nineteenth century) and 1950 (*see* Table 9-I)
underscore some of the vast changes that have taken place. The current time budget of work has changed little in the past thirty years.

A comparison of the work life of the average worker in the United
States was made from data prepared by Seymour Wolfbein. He
compared the number of man-years of lifetime work of cohorts born
in 1900 and 1960. "A group of 100,000 boys born alive and experiencing the mortality and labor force conditions existing today will put

211

Table 9-I

Time Budget of an Adult Worker (in hours)

| | TRADITIONAL EPOCH | | 1950 | |
	Daily	Annual	Daily	Annual
Sleep and Meals (365 days)	11	4,015	11	4,015
Leisure				
Sunday and Holidays				
(60 days)	-	780	-	780
Paid vacation (19 days)	-	-	-	182
Daily leisure time	-	-	3	873
Recesses in daily work	1	305	1	291
Journey to and from work	-	-	1	291
Work	12	3,660	8	2,328
Total hours	24	8,760	24	8,760
Leisure hours	-	780	-	1,835

Source: Fourastie, Jean: *The Causes of Wealth,* trans. by Theodore Caplow, Glencoe, Ill., The Free Press, 1960, p. 169. Copyright© by The Free Press. Reprinted by permission.

in about a million more man-years of work during their lifetimes than did their counterparts under 1900 conditions — an increase of almost one-third. A comparable group of girls today will almost triple the performance of their 1900 counterparts."[3]

These data reveal one of the basic elements in the three-fold rise in the gross national product, per capita, in the United States during the past half century.

Not only has longevity contributed to the increase in manpower potential and wealth, but it has also brought an increase in the time the average person spends outside of the labor force. Table 9-II shows that *"life, work-life, and years spent outside the labor force have all three increased for the population in recent years."*[4] The nine-year increase in years spent outside the labor force has been roughly divided between an increase in time spent in education and training, and retirement.

Also, the *work-life* for males has increased by another nine years. Despite this increase during the first half of the twentieth century, the proportion of life spent in the work force has declined with industrialization. The data from thirty-seven countries, classified by degree of industrialization, indicate that in fully industrialized countries, the average proportion of lifetime spent in the work force was

Table 9-II

Life and Working Life Expectancy in
the United States 1900-70 (In Years)

Year	MEN			WOMEN		
	Life Expect.	Work Life Expect.	Years Outside Labor Force	Life Expect.	Work Life Expect.	Years Outside Labor Force
1900*	48.2	32.1	16.1	50.7	6.3	44.4
1940	61.2	38.3	22.9	65.9	12.1	53.8
1950	65.5	41.9	23.6	71.0	15.2	55.8
1960	66.6	41.4	25.2	73.1	20.1	53.0
1970	67.1	41.1	26.0	74.8	22.9	51.9

*Data for 1900 are based on whites in death-registration states. Originally found in: Wolfbein, Seymour L.: Changing patterns of working life, (U.S. Department of Labor, Office of Manpower, Automation, and Training, August, 1963).

Source: Seymour L. Wolfbein: *Employment and Unemployment in the United States: A Study of the American Labor Force,* Chicago, Science Research Associates, 1964, p. 120. The 1970 data was provided by correspondence with the author.

65 percent, in semi-industrialized countries 67 percent, and 70 percent in agricultural countries.[5] These data are of limited utility when projected beyond the present.

A discussion of the hours and years of work-life has only become applicable with the modern-day delineation between work and non-work. In the tribal and early agrarian societies of the past, no such clear distinctions were made. The initial events that began to separate lifetime into a number of special categories of activity and social roles were the requirement of a certain period of formal education and the enactment of laws regulating the minimum age for workers. Both of these features in the chronology of life in modern society have delayed entry into the work force. Long life and increased productivity have made this possible and presumably desirable. The same is true for retirement.

Half a century ago, a man's working life was roughly equivalent to his expected length of life.[6] Since that time, the average number of years spent in retirement has more than doubled and is climbing. The relative certainty of retirement from work and the arbitrary timing of this important event have caused a number of problems. The present-day lack of the social roles and institutional developments needed to make an easy personal adjustment to retirement and old age are important aspects of contemporary social problems. An important element inherent in the problems of both retirement and the extension of education and training lies in the economic consequences of the changing age composition of society. Long life and low birth rates are the major factors.

The ability of a society to sustain the costs of a large and comprehensive educational structure and a disability and retirement system have become very strained. Fortunately, the rapid influx of married women into the labor force has offset some of the employment needs for countries experiencing these changes.

Spectacular control over the death of infants and children has freed the average woman from the need to spend a decade or more of intermittent pregnancies and childbearing. In addition to effective contraceptive methods and the changing norms governing the woman's role and function in society, long life has provided a large pool of potential workers.

Census data for the United States reveals the importance of women in the work force since 1890.[7] Participation of women in the labor force has more than doubled since the first census (participation rate of 18.2 percent in 1890 to 48.5 percent in 1977). The most striking change involves older women. They (45-64) have almost quadrupled their rate of participation in the labor force (1890 - 12.1; 1970 - 47.8). Men (45-64) declined from 92 to 87 percent during the same period. Older women account for over one third of the 40,067,000 women (45-64 years of age) in the labor force.[8] They have helped to take the place of retiring men. The increased withdrawal of men past fifty-five from the labor force has been offset by the growing tendency of older women to work during their middle years. The result is that even though men are retiring sooner than they once did, the percentage of jobholders in the adult population has remained quite constant.[9] Male and female trends in labor force participation seem to be reversing themselves. As the proportion of working women increases, the proportion of men declines. This phenomena is also reflected in the unemployment levels among middle-aged and older males. In 1977, 8.4 percent of all unemployed men in the United States were forty-five or over. In the category of long-term unemployed (27 weeks or more), 15.9 percent were in the older age-group.[10] The extent to which the trends will continue is impossible to predict. The recent changes in women's roles have yet to be fully felt throughout modern society.

The general conceptions of the work role and the perspectives affecting the relationships between aging, work, and retirement remain essentially those of the recent past. Age has generally been considered a deficiency in the otherwise efficient worker. The need for brawn, energy, and stamina in carrying out normal work functions was undeniable in the past. However, with the rapid increase of our service-dominated urban economy, most jobs demand neither brawn nor physical stamina, but rather, care and attention to detail, consistency and judgment. Though these qualities are not confined to the young, nor are they even at their peak among the young, the present-day cult of youth results in discrimination against the older worker.

Service related economic activities are expanding in the modern industrial countries. The corresponding work roles do not put a premium on physical prowess and energy; therefore, early retirement may turn out to be socially deleterious and economically costly. Present-day retirement ages, roughly set at age sixty-five, may be too late for heavy production work and occupations like coal mining, but for many professions, such as technical, executive, and coordinating positions, it may be too early. If, however, the apparent strong support for the forty-hour week remains unassailable, the current retirement ages may be necessary. The development of jobs appropriate for those who could work effectively during a twenty- to thirty-hour workweek would be of considerable help in solving some of the social and economic problems of the aged, youth, women with small children, and partially disabled. Although flexibility in retirement age and workweek are socially important in modern techonological society, income and the lack of social roles are also important issues in coping with the consequences of longevity and high level technology.

Facing these issues may demand a new system for determining who will become workers and nonworkers and under what conditions. As indicated, changes in the workweek regarding the utilization of part-time employment and variable retirement ages could have profound effects on the composition of the work force. This, in turn, would affect the distribution of income. However, certain economic facts compound the difficulty of dealing with these problem areas. One of these areas involves the productivity of labor in modern industrial economies. "Since men can produce more and more goods in fewer and fewer years, the problem is one of evening our lifetime earnings in such a way as to provide adequately for the young nonworking years and the years spent in retirement. The traditional scheme of distribution, which tends to make current participation in the labor force a condition of receiving income, will be altered within the present decade (the 1960s) primarily as a result of growing pressure to extend the period of education and training of young men."[11]

Although Kreps was correct in forecasting a change in distribution of income, she omitted an important element in the argument. That is, that productivity in modern society is highly variable. For example, the production of most material goods has shown an increase in productivity since the rise of industrialization. However, the output of services ranging from medical care, television repairs, police protection, and old age recreation do not exhibit the same upward productivity curves as the production of material goods. The importance of this difference is enhanced by the fact that "since World War II, services have constituted the fastest-growing area of the U.S. economy, rising to 157 percent between 1957 and 1970, compared with an increase of 119 percent for the economy as a whole."[12]

The attempts to improve productivity in the field of services, whether they are defined as economic or social, are difficult. For example, determining the appropriate level of efficiency and productivity of school teachers, social scientists, biologists, social workers, or policemen is extremely difficult. As might be expected, programs aimed at increasing the productivity of workers in these areas have had relatively little success. The optional size of school classes, productivity of scientists engaged in pure research, or the number and deployment of police needed to control crime are constantly debated. Indications are that many of the services needed in modern society cannot be done cheaply or be expected to follow the logic that the greater the number of units (often people) processed, the less it costs per unit. In some instances, the exact opposite may be true — for example, in education or crime prevention. A large school system usually implies a large urban population, which in turn, means variation or heterogeneity. A school system filled with students from a large range of family backgrounds will experience demands for a wide and diversified set of courses and learning activities. This requires the hiring of specially qualified teachers whose relative scarcity commands higher salaries.

Present conceptions of the life course and the structure of work and economics concentrates the period of paid work in the years of twenty to sixty-five. As Kreps noted, the distribution of income over the lifespan of the individual creates economic problems.[13] The normal earning period of the average person is limited to a proportionately shorter and shorter period of the life course. This has posed serious problems for the development of roles involving personal responsibility among the young and those that are defined as useful for the retired person. A large stumbling block in the development of social roles for the nonworking people is the importance of money as the major criterion of the value of a given task. Work done without pay is viewed as unimportant. That this criterion will be altered very much in the near future seems doubtful. This does not, however, preclude a decline in the symbolic importance of money. It means that it will remain as a significant criterion in the foreseeable future.[14]

At this time in the United States, distribution of income throughout the life course is affected by taxation, social security, and programs such as Job Corps and CETA. The major problems with the programs for the elderly are the lack of socially useful roles open to the people who participate and the inadequate incomes they receive. Providing useful roles probably will require provisions for new types of paid work. This is especially important for those workers who by age fifty-five find it difficult to keep up with the work demands of strenuous jobs. In underground mining, assembly line work, truck driving, and heavy day labor, early retirement is desirable for many men. At a retirement age of fifty-five, many men can expect to live about twenty years longer. Though some might desire work-free lives provided they had an adequate income, many others would welcome the chance for some kind of work.[15] How to provide such opportunities is one of the problems facing modern societies.

Careers and the Professions

The concepts of *career* and *profession* acquire full sociological meaning in the middle years of life in terms of longevity. At what point middle age begins and ends varies with the degree and tempo of social change. During the Romantic Era, a great many of the leading figures of the time seemed to mature early and reach the peak of their careers at a time that would now be considered a juvenile age. Many died before age fifty (Byron was 36), and a substantial number were dead before thirty. A great many of the productive men and women who died early would have lived into old age had they lived in the present period. They would have had long work careers.

The prolongation of life has particular relevance for the emergence of the concept of career. The use of this term in referring to a person's major occupational life is of relatively recent origin. One of the first instances of its use, in the present-day sense, is attributed to George Eliot in 1868.[16] The definition of career varies in the literature on the sociology of work. For our purposes, the most applicable definition is one that is somewhat restricted: "A career . . . is a succession of related jobs, arranged in a hierarchy of prestige, through which persons move in an ordered, predictable sequence."[17]

Wilensky estimated that, in 1960, only about a third or a fourth of the American labor force were following careers, though the proportion might be increasing.[18] "Although career workers comprise a minority of the work force, they are a major source of stability for modern society, as Weber, Mannheim, and many others have noted. Every group must recruit and maintain its personnel and motivate role performance. Careers serve these functions for organizations, occupational groups and societies. . . . 'By holding out the prospect of continuous, predictable rewards, careers foster a willingness to train and achieve, to adopt a long view and defer immediate gratification for the later payoff.' "[19]

Mannheim considered a bureaucratically organized society as a prerequisite to the development of careers. That is, careers can only emerge "in societies where the future is predictable, where the distribution of power is no longer a matter of dispute, and where some sort of plan can be made and executed on the basis of preexistent decisions."[20]

The definition of the work period as a career can only occur on a wide scale in a society that has become somewhat bureaucratically organized, nurtures a future-oriented life perspective, and has a minimum of living time in which to pursue a career. Before the time of increased longevity, men and women had shorter lives and a death-oriented perspective. Those who lived longer than average, however, became socially defined as old at a relatively early age. By past standards, a man of fifty was perceived as old.[21]

Long life makes it possible to seriously consider pursuing a career. It also contributes to the development of a stable social context within which high levels of individual achievement can be realistically contemplated and accomplished. This is particularly important for those of artistic, scientific, and scholarly careers that demand extensive education, long gestation periods, or the slow steady building of skills and knowledge.

The study of careers has led scholars to establish chronologies for those who follow careers. Miller and Form identify five stages in the work career. "The stages are: preparatory period (0-15 years of age); initial work period (15-18 years); trial work period (18-34); stable work periods (34-64 years); and retirement."[22]

Havighurst investigated role performance and the development of life-style in an aged population.[23] Utilizing cluster analysis, he was able to identify five major role clusters, each of which was characterized as a *life-style*. Although Havighurst's concept of life-style has a more general connotation than the concept of career, his findings are relevant to the present discussion. He reported that "a person's pattern of role performance or 'life-style' is established in early middle age, by the fifties, and tends to persist into the sixties."[24] Commenting on the work of Havighurst, Williams states that it "gives a picture of the period from forty to seventy as essentially a plateau in relation to the competence with which people perform social roles."[25]

In the context of longevity, career (or similar plateau in the life course) is of particular interest. Prior to the increase in life expectancy, relatively few lived much beyond the early years of the fifty- to seventy-year period. In contemporary society, the peak of many careers often occurs in the forty-five to sixty-year period and may even extend to age sixty and beyond, especially in careers involving political or administrative authority. Whether or not this plateau phenomenon is primarily a function of biological age and corresponding psychological factors or social structural features of the work environment is not fully known. If it is the latter, a change in social structure presumably may invalidate the notion of plateau as a feature of long life. Our earlier assumption, however, that the nature of modern industrial society (and the exigencies of long life) will continue to demand high levels of education and training coupled with trial and testing periods implies a necessity for rewards across the long term. Such rewards need not necessarily be pecuniary. Thus, the perception of the plateau as a pay-off period in the lives of career-oriented humans becomes important. It is a period during which we are somewhat assured of a stable work life and free from a capricious rise or fall in status, social well-being, or income. From this point of view, there seems little doubt that the prolongation of life forms one of the critical underpinnings of the development of those occupations that can be defined as careers.

The professions provide the most distinct examples of career occupations. They embody a high order of future orientation, involving extensive rational planning and organized activity, which is begun and perpetuated by long and meticulous education, training, and internship. A key feature in the contemporary development of the professions is the professional school.

The requirement that would-be professionals devote many years to formal education provides the opportunity for socialization, education, and training. Socialization of the student means that professional practices and behavioral codes can be more directly transmitted to the next generation. This helps maintain continuity in the traditions that constitute an important aspect of the know-how and protective armor of professional groups. Since the professional is primarily engaged in dispersing either rational, scientific, or traditional services of an important kind, he needs to develop protection from the consequences of error or failure. Some part of this protection rests on social solidarity and is buttressed by traditions and widely held norms of practice.

Strong traditions and powerful norms of professional conduct frequently inhibit changes in professional behavior. The prolongation of life insures that the professions will be comprised of a large proportion of older people, a change that has already occurred in some professional groups.

Although there are formal differences between a professional and a bureaucrat, both share a strong emphasis on continuity, stable relations, and formal norms of conduct. In his analysis of the evils of bureaucracy, Von Mises stated that "Young men are deprived of any opportunity to shape their own fate." The "only prospect is to start at the lowest rung of the bureaucratic ladder and to climb slowly in strict observance of the rules formulated by older superiors."[26]

In the past, the rarity of large numbers of older professionals affected the attitudes of younger members' towards them. In addition to long practice and experience, the informal influence and power of the successful older professional enhanced his or her prestige. This was particularly true when the number of professionals was much smaller, and they were known to each other within a city or region. Today, when professionals number in the thousands and include many persons with long experience, age-associated prestige is not inevitably forthcoming. The older established members of a given profession do, however, exercise a certain amount of control over the requirements for membership. Nontheless, new developments in the professional world may have begun to dilute some of the control held by those who serve as the gatekeepers.

A recent development basic to many professions, is the linking of professional practice with a burgeoning research activity. This tends to increase new knowledge and techniques at a rate that speeds up the obsolescence of those who have completed their formal training and are no longer closely affiliated with professional schools and research institutes. The continually shifting base of reliable knowledge on which the profession must rely serves as a powerful factor in initiating change within a profession.

The level of education and the awareness of the fluctuating nature of scientific knowledge held by many of their clients force the professional to rely on the expert or specialist whose function it is to translate the very latest knowledge into practice. In general, this situation has enhanced the importance of merit and scientific achievement and diminished the traditional type of authority based on age and experience. Some of this effect may be attributed to the rapid increase in knowledge and the extended length of professional training. The emergence of the expert puts a premium on specific knowledge and technical skills and has allowed the young to rise quickly on the basis of merit. This has curbed the power of the older nonspecialized professionals. After the transitional period has passed and the entire profession has shifted and developed all pertinent specialties, the older specialist may be able to build and maintain a strong position in determining the current conduct and future of the professional recruits. This may lead some to believe that the future favors conservatism for the professions.

This argument, however, lacks adequate support. The viewpoint fails to consider that conditions favoring a relatively high degree of dynamism have also developed within the professions. These conditions have resulted from a greater use of the scientific mode of inquiry, increases in knowledge and its consequences for education, and from the aforementioned emphasis placed on merit and achievement. The assumed conservatism of age is offset by the dynamism within the professional sphere. Ultimately, this dynamic process may alter the normative structure of the professions and help maintain a continuous sensitivity to new influences from within as well as without.

The modern professional's involvement is solving problems for an ever widening clientele within the society has meant a concomitant increase in prestige and material rewards for all professionals. This has been instrumental in attracting considerable talent to the professions. Talent is probably always a threat to traditional modes of behavior.

New and important roles for older professionals may add another dimension to long life and its relationship to the professions. Older professionals are often in a position to perform a unique service to a professional community, especially those who have been able to compete successfully with the younger and highly trained members. Role changes resulting from the division of labor in modern physics are indicative of such possibilities. A career in physics seems to divide itself into two distinct phases. The first calls for intensive research activity during young adulthood and early middle age; the second involves the managing and administering of research during and after middle age.[27]

The sciences are characterized by variations in roles resulting from what Glaser calls "comparative failure in science."[28] Since the scientific community places considerable emphasis on attaining recognition, the feeling of comparative failure is ever present. Eminent men are the role models for other scientists, but the nature of the scientific community makes it inevitable that most scientists will not be able to fully emulate their idols.[29] With increased longevity, more of a given cohort of new scientists will live to experience and be forced to adjust to feelings of comparative failure.

Glaser notes, however, that there are degrees of failure. Scientists who are accorded an average amount of recognition as compared to those who receive less recognition seem to function more adequately in their field. The need for large numbers of undistinguished scientists are factors in developing the institutional patterns that allow the "comparative failure to harbour feelings of modest and limited success." Although an important factor in the development of the newer roles and statuses in contemporary science is the tremendous rise in the number of scientists, a longer and more active life has also contributed to the change in career patterns.

Although seniority in a profession is of declining importance as a prime criterion of status, the growing number of retired individuals, e.g. partners of law firms, professors emeritus, physicians and surgeons, clergymen, and teachers have important implications for the future of the professions.[30] Placing retired or semiretired professionals in such influential positions as members of college boards of trustees, research policy review boards, publication boards, and high-level consultative positions in government and industry represents an important effect of longevity. Relatively good health and the postponement of death make it probable that the older, prominent professionals will remain professionally active long after official retirement. If the retirement age remains the same or is lowered, a new status and corresponding role of the partially retired professional may emerge. If the income levels of professionals continue to rise, a greater variation in the timing of retirement will undoubtedly occur. Increased wealth will allow some to elect semiretirement at an earlier age than is now customary. It is already true for dentists.

Second Careers, Orderly Work Lives, and Longevity

Modern society and long life has not only influenced the development of careers, but it has also increased the possibilities of people deliberately making important changes during the course of a lifetime. Such factors as occupational obsolescence, dislocations resulting from social and economic change, career completion, the desire for interesting and socially useful work, and job dissatisfaction can present new opportunities if one can anticipate a long, and healthy life. The intensity of those factors that push and pull toward second careers is greatly increased with the prolongation of life. A life perspective that includes the recognition of the fact that life is both long and varied would tend to foster a consideration of the desirability of changing careers. Such consideration may be supported by the possibility that a career change may mean an increase in status, a potential for upward mobility, greater income, and job security.

Whatever effects long life has on the frequency and desirability of second careers, it occurs in middle age. A life perspective conducive to the willingness and ability to make fundamental changes in one's life appears to have its foundation in family background and education. Though career change most directly affects middle-aged participants, the development of new norms and values fostering the adoption of second careers will have an effect on old age as well. For persons who have stepped out of the ranks and followed new paths, old age will frequently be viewed much more favorably. Many of the attitudes of old people are determined by the events of their earlier life. For many, a life of some variety, which has involved risks and new opportunities, is much more likely to be viewed positively than a narrow and conventional existence in a single-stranded occupational career. Second careers developed in middle age by a large number of Americans provide evidence of the adaptability of men and women, as well as the potentialities of long life. The existence of many people who have changed their lives by new careers provide the examples needed to bring forth a new perspective of life.

The pursuit of second careers is common among certain occupational categories, for example, athletes, airline pilots, fashion models, military and police personnel, and housewives. One study done in the United States found that second career phenomenon to be the most common among contemporary married women. Over two-thirds of the group studied had previously been in business or professional occupations.[31]

The prolongation of life has not only contributed to the possibility of a second career, but to the general phenomena of an *orderly career*. The concept of orderly career has been used to describe an important aspect of work life. Wilensky defines the orderly career as one characterized by an orderly vertical progression in which "at least half the years covered in the work history are in jobs that are functionally related and arranged in a hierarchy of prestige, and the mobility pattern cuts across occupational strata."[32] Under this definition, many current work lives exhibiting second careers would be defined as orderly.[33] The majority of the work force in modern societies spend their lives in a disorderly or chaotic pattern of jobs. The distinction between orderly and chaotic careers may be important. Wilensky's research findings indicate that orderliness may have serious consequences for nonwork aspects of the social order:

> Orderly experience, in the economic system is associated with many social ties which range broadly and at the same time overlap. Men who have predictable careers for at least a fifth of their worklives belong to more organizations, attend more meetings, and average more hours in organizational activity. Their attachments to the local community are also stronger — indicated by support of local schools and, to a lesser extent, by contributions to church and charity.
>
> In both formal and informal contacts, the men of orderly career, more than their colleagues of chaos, are exposed to a great variety of people: the fellow-members they see in clubs and organizations represent many social and economic levels; frequently seen relatives and close friends are more scattered in space both social and geographical, cutting across neighborhoods, workplace, occupations, or income brackets. Finally the total participation pattern of the orderly is more coherent: close friends tend to form a circle, and they overlap work contacts. (The data do not support the view that best friends share voluntary association memberships.) There is some indication that these friendships, anchored in workplace, forming a leisure-time clique, may also be longer lasting.[34]

The prolongation of life has increased the probability that a great many men and women will experience disorderly or chaotic work lives. Even though life expectancy after midlife has not increased a great deal since the middle of the nineteenth century, the number of aged in the population has increased significantly. Thus, the impact of disorderly worklives has increased.

If orderliness is a desirable goal, it may necessitate the institutionalization of second careers for most of the work force — if some measure of disorderliness can be eliminated from the first part of the work life. Orderly careers characterized by spending one's entire work life within one specific occupation or company organization is probably a type of career orderliness that modern industrial society cannot afford. The institutionalization of second careers, with the aim of achieving a minimal degree of orderliness, demands a number of basic changes in the social psychological and economic conditions governing work in modern society. The concept of orderliness may have to be broadened to include stability in work groupings, general working conditions and a stable income over the entire work life. If a minimal income and the assurance that some kind of work was always available were institutionalized, the consequences of chaotic and disorderly work lives would probably not be as important as Wilnesky's data indicate. This could facilitate a greater concern over the type of occupation one pursues.

An awareness of increased longevity can mean that finding the right occupation becomes a powerful norm for increasing numbers of people and that remaining in a job that one dislikes becomes morally reprehensible. Furthermore, the critical evaluations placed on occupation as the criterion of a person's worth may diminish in importance with the adaptation to a long and healthy life. With the potentiality of having several occupations during one's lifetime that perhaps vary in status, the importance of occupational status might decline. Other criteria such as education, life-style, income, or notoriety would be enhanced.

Social Aspects of Retirement and Long Life

A great deal has been written about old age in the past few years, and the most salient subject has been retirement from gainful employment. An important aspect of these writings has been to report on the social and psychological consequences of retirement.

In past times, a few men lived long enough to retire from work since life became settled enough to sustain them in food and clothing, but only in recent times has retirement become expected and commonplace.[35] Geoffrey Gorer has commented that "retirement, as a normal expectation, is an unparalleled development in human life and human history; it poses problems which no society before the twentieth century has had to try to solve."[36] "I know of no other situation which has no analogues either in the past or in the less developed areas of the contemporary world."[37]

The study of retirement has uncovered a substantial number of myths. One of these myths shows that retirement has a deleterious effect on mental and physical health. It has been over twenty years since several studies found this to be true.[38] There is, of course, no doubt that the act of retiring from full-time work represents a major life change, a change that points to the fact that death is a step closer. Personal identification with one's work and retirement income determine the degree to which retirement becomes problematic and thus defined as a depressing end.

One of the social contradictions of modern times is that in a society that "is able to support an increasing porportion of nonproductive members, we are faced with the fact that all of the values of the society are directed at the glorification of economic roles . . . , and in general at the activities related to youth. Hence we have the crux of the sociopsychological problem of retirement."[39] The extent and nature of the problem varies a great deal with the circumstances of retirement. Such are the circumstances of whether or not the decision to retire is voluntary or forced.

Although the life course involves a succession of role changes, most of the changes are made by passing through recognized transitional periods that allow anticipatory socialization to take place. A certain amount of preparation for each new role occurs. However, "the retirement role is beset with a lack of socially defined appropriate behavior inasmuch as it also lacks a clearly defined social position in the structure of society. In one sense, retirement is a negation of the traditional values surrounding the place of work in Western society and men are loath to surrender the identifying position in society which a job bestows."[40]

The Western ethic of work as the principal measure of the value of the individual and the *raison d'être* for life itself has contributed much to the negative attitudes associated with retirement. The most extreme manifestation of the deleterious effect of retirement is based on the belief that leaving one's work is tantamount to being thrown on society's ash heap, equivalent to social death. In the recent past, the assumption often was made that social death was quickly followed by biological death. Mortality data indicates that persons who are forced into compulsory retirement have no higher death rate than would be expected for their age-group. Those who retire voluntarily have a higher rate than expected, which is probably due to the fact that a considerable number of them retired because of advanced age and ill health.[41] Streib and Schneider state that health declines with age but not with retirement, and unskilled workers showed a small improvement in health after retirement.[42]

The importance of work in the life of modern man is hard to over-estimate. This is particularly true since work and leisure have become distinctly defined and call for separate role behavior. Since work has become such an important indicator of status and life-style as well as the basis for material security, abrupt retirement can have detrimental effects. Tartler comments that ". . . work is the principle source of social contacts on which even private social activities frequently depend. . . . A man finds in his work a primary, if not the only, reliable interpretative medium in a world that is steadily becoming more complicated and anonymous. . . ."[43] With the high level of specialization and complexity of contemporary modern life, "work has the social function of coordinating and confining the uncontrollable and intricate possible human activities to a more-or-less limited system of actions, and work thus plays an important role in helping the individual master life, even if it is felt to be a burden. In this way, work functions as a relief because it helps a man establish himself in his environment through continuity of action in an occupational structure which is circumscribed by relatively constant means and goals. Thus the environment is stabilized and the worker himself is stabilized in it."[44] Also, much of what constitutes the individual's personality and self-image is intimately tied to the sphere of work.

An important feature in the ideology of work is the major criterion of value or usefulness, which is measured in monetary terms. This is a guiding principle through the greatest part of the life course and does not readily change in old age. Fried found that elderly, lower-class persons did not consider activities culturally acceptable unless they were deemed useful, and the criterion of usefulness was a monetary reward.[45] Nonetheless, there is impressionistic evidence from many elderly people that unpaid volunteer work is increasing and gaining favor as an optional form of useful activity after retirement.

The commonly held concept of retirement fails to fit the circumstances resulting from the great increase in longevity. Retirement is viewed at its worst with the loss of one's central role in life and at its best as a period of free time in which to pursue pleasurable activities. These two alternative conceptions portray the end of life in a much too simple fashion. They obscure and diminish the importance of other roles that do not end with retirement from work. Some of these roles gain importance in our world of affluence and long life, such as the roles of active citizen, consumer, spouse, parent, and friend. Though it is only beginning, there is evidence that a rational concern with citizen and consumer participation is on the rise. The interpersonal relationships of marital, parental, and friendship roles are enhanced by increased self-awareness and the study of psychology and sociology. The various encounter groups, sensitivity sessions, and how-to-do-it books also attest to the concern regarding interpersonal relationships during the life course.

If retirement were viewed more as a process of changing social relationships than a loss of something very important, a perspective conducive to successful long life could more readily develop. The process of retirement is, in fact, never finished. Like one's earlier life, it involves continual change and adaptation.

Although the negative connotation of retirement seems to be declining in the United States, the same is not true for all industrialized countries. A comparative study indicated that British and Danish retirees are less likely to enjoy retirement than Americans.[46] A study done at the University of Chicago that matched groups of older and younger workers recorded attitudes toward retirement. Everyone expected to retire. The younger men favored early retirement, whereas many who were closer to retirement did not wish to.[47] The data further revealed that the younger men were the most unrealistic about the possibilities of life in retirement. Most men have probably accepted the fact that they will live long enough to experience retirement. The educational process, however, and the development of a perspective that fully recognizes a long life consisting of an adequate life outside of an economically productive role have not fully emerged.

The choice of whether to work or retire may be determined by fewer people as more and more firms merge into large conglomerates. Currently, that portion of the older population who do not work for large corporations are the ones who most frequently decide to work beyond the normal retirement age.

Since the 1890s, those who worked in the primary sector of the economy (those engaged in agriculture, fishing, and mining) and in the tertiary sector (those providing services, professional, and otherwise) were the ones who worked beyond the official retirement age. Workers in the secondary or manufacturing sector have had the earliest average age at retirement. This sector and the primary sector of agriculture, fishing and mining have decreased in proportion to the total work force.

These trends are continuing. As agriculture moves into the new green revolution of agri-genetics, the number of independent farmers will probably decrease even further. The required technology is very costly. "The new superproducts manufactured by Du Pont and Monsanto may only be affordable by the 3 percent of farmers who account for 40 percent of all sales of farm goods."[48] The large capital requirements of this second green revolution could put more farmers into the ranks of corporate industrial workers.

The change towards corporate organization in fishing that has taken place in Japan and the Soviet Union may portend the future for the fishing industry in the United States. In contrast to agriculture and fishing, retirement age in mining has been lowered through the efforts of the United Mine Workers.

Further developments in the centralization of control over the conditions of work may have important consequences for the increased number of elderly. With greater centralization, the choice of working beyond age sixty-five (and now seventy) may not be made by the individual concerned, but by government and corporate policy makers.

Over the past decade or two, many have chosen early retirement, that is, before age sixty-five. This trend may be changing, according to a recent estimates.[49] The financial consequences of high inflation appear to be an important basis for the increases in retirement age in some sectors of the economy. Improvements in the education and health of older Americans and the increase in age from sixty-five to seventy for mandatory retirement also have influenced retirement age. Furthermore, the Department of Health and Welfare has suggested raising the retirement age for Social Security to sixty-eight years of age. The basic reasoning behind this suggestion is that it would help prevent future insolvency for the Social Security fund. This suggestion has been challenged by many gerontologists on the grounds that it would work many hardships for certain workers. Many workers retire before sixty-five for health reasons.

Raising the age of retirement, however, by changing the Social Security regulations or making it easier for older workers to stay in the work force could be socially and psychologically beneficial. Flexible work schedules, reduced work weeks, job changes to fit health problems, or monetary inducements such as increased social security benefits for later retirement might raise the age of retirement and have an effect in delaying the onset of old age. At present, retirement tends to signal the beginning of old age. Any delay in retirement age for the mass of American workers could change the definition of old age and some of the attitudes and expectations toward those in the later years. The replacement of most mandatory retirement rules with criteria based on ability to function would direct attention away from chronological age. Also, since attitudes toward others are somewhat contingent on occupational roles, many more of the elderly who were still working would retain their place as full-fledged citizens. Since retired people hold a special place in society and are not as highly valued as working people, later retirement would have positive effects on the status of the elderly.

Longevity and the Economics of Retirement and Leisure

As we have indicated, retirement from work is a new phenomenon; it was relatively uncommon before 1900. The difference between life expectancy and work life expectancy at that time was only three years.[50] Or stated in another way, by 1900, more than two thirds of all men age sixty-five and over were gainfully employed. This proportion had dropped to 32.2 percent by 1960, and fell to 24.8 percent by 1970.[51]

Longevity has made retirement normal rather than exceptional, and the changeover has created many difficulties for those experiencing long life: ". . . , before 1940, only a privileged few could seriously look forward to a life in retirement which did not mean becoming dependent on family, kin, or friends, public assistance, or private charity. For the vast majority, retirement was a dreaded period signifying the end of social usefulness. . . ."[52] Though retirement has now become commonplace in modern societies, it is nevertheless fraught with ambiguity. In most societies, it is further complicated by the social psychological crisis of the loss of occupational role and decline in income.

Longevity is one of the causes of income problems for the retiree. Usually income drops substantially upon retirement. The longer one lives, the greater becomes the disparity between retirement income and income from work. At age sixty-five, the average married man in the United States can expect to live about fourteen more years, and his wife who may be a year or two younger will have almost twenty years left to live. Should there be a lowering of retirement age or an increase in life expectancy, (both are possibilities), a married couple could have two decades of nonworking life.[53] Present economic trends indicate that "during these twenty years, dramatic changes are likely to occur in the income position of persons remaining in the labor force. If the economy's real rate of growth were as high as 4 percent annually, the total output of goods and services would roughly double in two decades. Working persons and their families would thus enjoy a 100 percent increase in real income, while the bulk of retirees continued to live on incomes that were fixed. To the extent that prices rose, the aged's income position would be worsened even further."[54] Under such conditions, long life is scarred by poverty or, at best, serious economic restrictions. The socioeconomic issue in all of this is, how can the retirement years be freed from these economic facts?

Under current American economic ideology, the issue leads to the problem of smoothing out or apportioning work life income over the whole lifespan rather than bunching it in the working years of twenty to sixty-five, and leaving roughly twenty problematic years at the end of life.[55] Viewed in this manner, the problem becomes one involving the distribution of work and nonwork time or leisure over the life course. In this regard, Kreps advances a theory of human satisfaction. She states

> it is a balancing of goods (i.e., income) and leisure that maximizes satisfactions, and this balance may be disturbed by too much free time in one stage of life and too little in another. Similarly, a somewhat more even distribution of income throughout the lifespan might increase the total utility of any given amount of lifetime earnings. Such a smoothing of income can be and often is accomplished by individual savings arrangements; many people, on the other hand, have extremely high time preferences for goods and relatively little willpower for saving. Reliance on some form of forced savings is therefore quite common.[56]

Goods and services produced in one year cannot be stored for later use, for example, during retirement. Savings or annuities are only deferred claims, and hence subject to variation in the purchasing power of money over time. In recent times, inflation has plagued many of those on fixed incomes in the United States. The solution to the income maintenance problem, according to Kreps, would be facilitated by the smoothing of lifetime earnings, and this in turn, could more readily be accomplished by a longer work life; that is, spreading leisure time throughout the work life rather than bunching it in the retirement period.

In favoring changes in the social norms governing retirement, Kreps cites information on retirement in European countries: "Although the European nations, with lower incomes and less free time, do not face this question immediately, it is evident that reduction in retirement age has a very low priority in their range of leisure preferences, which are for shorter workweeks, additional holidays in some cases, and extended education and training periods."[57] She further states that many American workers might also prefer a shorter workyear if they were given a choice. In Australia, the labor unions long ago opted for more leisure in lieu of pay.[58]

A number of large American labor unions, however, have been successful in negotiating a lowering of retirement ages for their members. The United Mine workers succeeded in lowering retirement age from sixty to fifty-five. The United Auto Workers lowered the ages from sixty-five to sixty. An official of the Teamsters has stated that retirement at age fifty-seven is " 'almost a physical necessity' for truck drivers."[59] If retired truck drivers are comparable to the average American male, they have almost two decades of retirement living. In 1978, the life expectancy for fifty-seven year-old males was seventy-six years, or nineteen years after retirement at age fifty-seven.[60] Despite attempts to move towards early retirement on the part of large industrial unions, retirement age tends to be affected by the condition of the labor market. A softening of the demand for labor and increased unemployment are major stimulants in promoting early retirement.

Although retirement age is frequently tied to actuarial considerations and the economic conditions in a particular industry or even the labor market as a whole, the trend has been to eliminate mandatory retirement age. Arguments favoring a fixed retirement age prevailed for several decades, but since January 1979, amendments to the Age Discimination Act raised the age of compulsory retirement from sixty-five to seventy. In 1981, the White House conference on aging voted to eliminate mandatory retirement.

In light of variations in health, working conditions, needs and desires for income, and personal life-styles, the most logical approach to the question of retirement age is one that embodies maximum flexibility. One such system, which has served as model for some private companies, covers employees of the U.S. federal government. This system allows one to retire as early as fifty-five years, while allowing others to continue until age seventy.

The major difficulty in early retirement lies in the income provisions of most pension plans. Under present circumstances in the United States, the only prospect for early retirement lies in the expansion and improvement of private pension plans. Although there has been a large expansion in private pensions, a minority of persons benefit substantially from these programs. Furthermore, most pension programs, in order to minimize cost, are calculated on a basis of late retirement, at least sixty-five and frequently older, except in those cases where very powerful unions have negotiated early retirement provisions. Since most employees under private pension systems do not have a vested right to money invested by both the company and the employee, frequent job changes and unemployment result in inadequate pension for thousands of workers.

The necessity for income maintenance over a long period of retirement demands provisions for pension programs that provide fully vested pension rights, either public or private. Under a system of vested rights to monies placed in pension funds, an individual would not be forced to remain with one employer, irrespective of working conditions or personal needs and desires. In effect, one could carry (portability) pension rights from one job to another. In addition, the fear of losing pension rights by having one's job terminated before the minimum age of retirement would be diminished.

For most of our history, private pension plans offered little or no protection for employees. Before the new law that required some form of vested pension funds, an Assistant Secretary of Labor stated "*If* you remain in good health, and *if* you stay with the same company until you are sixty-five, and *if* the company is still in business, and *if* your department has not been abolished, and *if* your job has not been made technologically obsolete, and *if* you have not been laid off too long a time, and *if* there is sufficient money, in the fund, you will get your pension."[61] An equitable set of private pension plans would have considerable impact on the lives of the aged.

Another serious issue for the aged is the problem of housing. The increased number of elderly has added new dimensions to the housing of modern populations. The desire for small, safe, and efficient housing units and the need for several levels of partial to full-care types of living accommodations have stimulated the development of a new housing market in the United States. This is particularly evident in the building of vast housing developments for the aged in the warmer climates of the southern and western areas of the country. The most recent surge in such housing accommodations is the establishment of various types of nursing homes.

In 1970, it was reported that the nursing home industry was one of the fastest growing sectors of the American economy.[62] At that time, approximately forty companies had announced plans to build and operate nursing homes, and 340 million dollars had been collected by selling stock to the public. This impending growth was on top of an already existent boom in nursing homes. Between 1966 and 1970, the number of nursing homes rose from 12,000 to 24,000. By 1970, new homes were opening at the rate of three per day.[63] The New York *Times* reported that the nursing home industry took in 2.5 billion dollars in 1969 and that two of every three dollars came from public sources. The recent boom in this segment of the housing and service area of the economy is largely due to the increasing consequences of long life and the federal financing of homes and facilities through Medicare and other programs.

Longevity itself has produced a large group of potentially infirm people. Of the twenty million or more Americans over sixty-five, a third of them are seventy-five years or older. The boom in nursing homes and other housing that is specifically designed and marketed to elderly people is another feature of modern industrial economies that has resulted from long life. The early development of large communities in Florida, Arizona, New Mexico, and California that have been exclusively planned for the aged have proved desirable for many elderly. Attempts to mix housing for the elderly with conventional housing is being attempted in planning new housing areas. The need for adequate housing for the elderly is intensified by the important changes that have affected the elderly population.

A large proportion of the elderly wish to live separately and independently from their children; small, but complete, housing units are needed. The prolongation of life also increases the need for hospital, infirmary, and nursing home space. Children of aged and infirm-aged parents do not usually have room to house an elderly parent, and also they lack the facilities for giving the kind of care frequently needed by the very old. Over the next twenty years, the number of elderly people over seventy-five will probably increase by approximately 53 percent, and those over eighty-five by 64 percent. It is this growing segment of the elderly population that will require specialized housing and health facilities.

Family, Work, and Retirement

Although the education-work-retirement pattern of life predominates among many Americans, there is a growing dissatisfaction with it, and some people attempt to break the sequence by changing careers. The new concepts of second career, midlife career shift, and flexible life scheduling all testify to the rising incidence of variations and alternatives to the traditional career approach.[64] Long life gives these new approaches a utility that is barely apparent at present.

It appears that second careers and flexible work schedules that fit the physical limitations of late middle age might help increase life satisfaction at the older ages. A perspective towards work that includes more than one occupation during a lifetime might allow a better adjustment between occupation and individual circumstance and thereby be more satisfactory over a longer life. Evidence indicates that those who like their work do not desire early retirement unless they have definite plans for other work or demanding avocational pursuits. If occupations later in life could be changed to fit the social psychological and physiological circumstances of late middle age and early old age, retirement would seem less compelling. Including adequate time for education and leisure throughout the work life would enhance these possibilities and reduce the sharp distinction existing between education, work, and leisure — a distinction that has done much to promote early retirement.

Retirement requires a change in identity that is similar to that associated with the facts of aging. Laufer and Bengtson state, "The emerging . . . period between disengagement from the identity built around the occupational-parental experience and the period before death becomes imminent is a place for renewing interests left dormant during middle adulthood: finding new interests, validating or reviewing past commitments, and above all establishing new facets of identity which will sustain a valued sense of self outside of the occupational-parental sphere."[65] The ideal of lengthening the period of work by discouraging early retirement does not alter or deny the validity of the above statement, but changes the timing of it.

The potentiality for making changes in the scheduling of education, work, and retirement along the life course is much more possible than making changes in the parent-family portion of life. The transition and identities related to work are open to greater experimentation and variety than are parental ones. This implies a need for public policies that deal directly with scheduling education, work, and retirement to conform to the realities of a long and healthy life. Occupational and career changes in later years need not result in feelings of loss. The lack of a second option or a repeat performance of the family roles does not necessarily apply to the work roles. Long life has, in effect, required changes in two important self-identities during the postparental and retirement periods — worker and parent. Some of these changes are affected by improved health among the elderly.

The increase in healthy life expectancy has altered and may continue to alter the timing of the changes traditionally thought to be associated with the years after sixty-five. "There are . . . important indications that the degenerative effects of aging are declining for the average person . . . , average life expectancy at age sixty-five has increased some 3.5 years between 1930 and 1976. Additionally, the health of the older person appears to be increasing. HEW data show that 'healthy life expectancy' has grown faster than overall life expectancy since 1958, with the average number of days of reported sickness a year for persons over sixty-five declining from 47.3 in 1958 to 38.0 in 1974."[66] This may partially be accounted for by the fact that work is becoming less physically demanding — another factor that may extend work life.

The emerging awareness that aging results in only slight losses in critical mental abilities and that exercise and medical intervention can maintain a relatively high level of physical capability over a long life provides greater options for the elderly. Furthermore, the fact that older workers are generally more productive than younger ones bodes well for making changes in work schedules in the older years.[67] These developments make the current debate regarding the proposal for increasing the official retirement age to sixty-eight much more realistic.

Economic Consequences of Cohort Size

The marked prolongation of life accompanying industrialization has changed the size of many of the birth cohorts in the overall age composition of modern societies. That is, a given birth cohort moving through the life course experiences the depletion of its numbers at a slower rate than formerly. Fluctuations in the economic situation will affect a larger proportion of those people who share membership in the same birth cohort than formerly when death would have eliminated many more of each cohort as they progressed through the life course. The lengthening of life means that a birth cohort remains larger and lasts longer. In turn, if the conditions of life become hazardous or crisis ridden for a particular cohort, the impact upon it would become more evident in the social, political, and economic life of the overall population. The size of a group that suffers misfortune from social and economic change is important in terms of the scope and magnitude of the social problems that result. However, the direct consequences for individuals or families of unemployment, war, epidemics, or other disruptive phenomena may be similar whether their numbers are large or small.

The cohort that contributes most heavily to a declining economic activity will suffer most and thus determine the nature of the social problem by virtue of the particular characteristics of the cohort effected. When, for example, the economic base in an area begins to decline, as was apparent in the coal and iron producing areas of the United States during the 1950s and 60s, the affected birth cohorts in the labor force were compelled to respond to the changing circumstances.

For example, in the iron mining areas of midwestern United States, the quality of the iron ore declined after almost half a century of intensive mining. In order to utilize the low grade ore, a high level of mechanization was introduced. The result was a radical decline in the number of workers needed to process the iron ore. This meant that several cohorts in the mining work force were drastically affected. At the time this occurred (late 1950s and 1960s), a large cohort of men aged forty to fifty-five were at a point in the life course when they had half-grown families and homes that were only partially paid for. Unemployment, the loss of a home, or forced early retirement from work had a profound impact on the families, as well as the communities involved. In some places, the younger families who wanted to leave and find work in other parts of the country could not find buyers for their houses. Some locked their houses and left, and others virtually gave them away.[68] Some elected to stay and go on the welfare rolls with the possibility of occasionally getting part-time or marginal jobs.

Under such conditions, the future of the community was shaped by disproportionately large numbers of people who were both aged and poor. The need to educate the young for a life away from their home community and provide welfare funds, medical facilities, and institutions for the aging became major social and economic problems for the area in question.

In terms of longevity, this example illustrates how crucial events can influence whole cohorts, even to the extent that premature loss of their major economic roles would speed up the onset of retirement and old age.

Historically one can speculate on the impact of severe economic decline on a community in 1700. The conditions of life and the life expectancy at the time determined that the forty to fifty-five year old cohorts were proportionately much smaller than in our American example from the 1950s and 60s. High death rates from infancy on would have depleted all eighteenth century cohorts in contrast to contemporary times.

The following table (Table 9-III) helps to illustrate this point. The proportion of the eighteenth century French cohorts surviving to age forty had been seriously depleted by age twenty, and continued at about the same rate to age sixty. Of the 502 survivors at age twenty, only 369 were still alive at age forty, and by age sixty only 214 of the original 1,000 had survived. In contrast, the cohorts in modern France suffered relatively modest losses. At age twenty, 940 had survived, at age forty, there were 901, and at sixty years, 754 of the 1,000 were still alive.

Table 9-III

Survival in 18th and 20th Century France
(Number of Survivors)

Age	France 18th Century	France 1958
Birth	1,000	1,000
1 year	767	960
20 years	502	940
40 years	369	901
60 years	214	754
80 years	35	298

Source: Adapted from a table in Sauvy, Alfred: *Fertility and Survival,* New York, Criterion Books, 1961, p. 43.

Under conditions of long life in modern industrial society, a cohort or set of cohorts adversely affected by economic circumstances continue to live on. Though the depletion rate for a contemporary cohort increases with age, the difference is substantial when compared to the past. Therefore, the problems faced by a large cohort in the midst of their work life, continues to ramify throughout the social structure.

One response to this has been the development of massive national programs to meet the problems of the large cohorts moving into old age. Many of these have found themselves without a means of livelihood or the financial ability to avail themselves of the prevailing medical services. Consequently, old age social insurance and Medicare have been instituted in the United States; the former was enacted in the depths of the Great Depression.

The increased number in the older cohorts have affected the level of awareness of problems and created an indirect and serious demand for both economic and political change.

Youth has traditionally been viewed as a potent force in revolutionary change. One reason for this is that the youthful cohorts in past populations were often proportionately large compared to those in middle and old age. Long life has, in some instances, changed the numerical balance. Middle-aged and old people now outnumber youth in certain time periods. It has been argued that youth have an ability to see problems and inconsistencies in traditional life-styles and modus operandi. In addition, they may be willing to take high risks. These characteristics may, however, be a result of social and cultural circumstances rather than an inherent capability of youthfulness. The variation in size of successive cohorts as they change over time may be of critical importance.

Joan Waring, in a study of the consequences of variation in the size of cohorts, states "It would seem that membership in a large cohort increases the motivation for deviance and membership in a small cohort increases the commitment to conformity."[69] She illustrates this with reference to the large cohorts of the 1960s and the small ones of the 1950s. Reference is made to the differences in allegiance to the *cohort flow process* of these contrasting cohorts. The cohort flow process refers to flow or movement of new cohorts into the social roles of preceding cohorts.

When a cohort is either much larger or smaller then the cohort it is destined to replace, the result is disordered cohort flow. That is, "the cohort is . . . simply too large or too small relative to the role spaces available to the age stratum."[70] Waring points out that dropping out phenomenon of the late 1960s was indicative of the deviance of a proportion of these youthful cohorts. Their motivation to drop out was a result of the recognition that the social rewards for conformity were at best uncertain and the competition for them keen. There were more young people than socially valued roles for the age group."[71] In contrast, the smaller cohorts of the 1950s found themselves in a flourishing economy with incentives that induced them to commit themselves to the system. Waring hypothesizes "that when the rewards for conformity are ample and easily accessible to an age stratum, the motivation for deviance is weakened."[72]

Variation in cohort size can reach such a degree that the flow from one age stratum to another is disrupted. "Moreover, we might predict that members of cohorts which typically disrupt the people-role balance may have, over their life course, a greater propensity for criminality, mental illness, drug abuse, and so on. Conversely, other cohorts may be remarkable for their conformity."[73] Cohort size can apparently be a powerful agent in affecting social change. Although the youth cohorts of the 1950s and 1960s did not owe their variation in size to high rates of death and disaster, the argument developed by Waring may be applicable to the earlier periods when death was pervasive at all age levels.

Middle-age cohorts of large size, and hence of political and economic power, are capable of exercising considerable pressure for social change. It was not youth or the aged that were instrumental in the enactment of social security. It was the middle-aged. The same can be said for the movement toward medical insurance for the elderly.

These and many other economic consequences have some of their roots in the population changes resulting from the prolongation of life. Since many of the changes have been taking place over an extended period in present-day industrial countries, the exact relationship of the various aspects of longevity are difficult to disentangle. Newly developing countries of the world, however, may serve as a natural experiment. Studies should be done of the impact of mortality change, the social policies that emerge in response to the expanded size, and the political and economic importance of certain cohorts in these populations.

REFERENCES AND NOTES

1. Fourastié, Jean: *The Causes of Wealth,* Glencoe, Ill., The Free Press, 1960, pp. 164-65.
2. *Ibid.,* p. 164.
3. Wolfbein, Seymour L.: *Employment and Unemployment in the United States: A Study of the American Labor Force,* Chicago, Science Research Associates, 1964, p. 121.
4. *Ibid.,* p. 120.
5. Kreps, Juanita M.: *Lifetime Allocation of Work and Leisure,* Washington, D.C., Social Security Administration, Research Report No. 22, 1968, p. 10.
6. That is, expected length of life at age fifteen.
7. U.S. Bureau of Census *Historical Statistics of the United States,* Colonial Times to 1970, Washington, D.C., p. 132; and U.S. Department of Labor, Bureau of Labor Statistics, *Handbook of Labor Statistics,* Bulletin #2000, 1979, Washington, D.C., U.S. Government Printing Office, 1979.
8. U.S. Department of Labor, Bureau of Labor Statistics, *Handbook of Labor Statistics,* Bulletin #2000, 1979, Washington, D.C., U.S. Government Printing Office, 1979.
9. *Ibid.,* pp. 24-27.
10. *Ibid.,* pp. 202-204.
11. Kreps, Juanita: Economic implications of shortened worklife, in P. From Hansen (Ed.) *Age With a Future,* Philadelphia, F.A. Davis Co., 1964, p. 508.
12. *The McGraw-Hill Dictionary of Modern Economics: A Handbook of Terms and Organizations,* New York: McGraw-Hill, 1973, p. 533.
13. A reminder may be in order. There is considerable difference between the distribution of income at a particular time and such issues as the redistribution of accumulated wealth or the control of wealth. Kreps seems to be mainly concerned with the former.
14. This issue was discussed in more detail in Chapter 8, Class, Status, and Long

Life.

15. Rose, Charles I. and Mogey, John M.: Aging and preference for later retirement. *Aging and Human Development, 3*:45ff, 1972; Institute of Gerontology: Older workers and retirement. *Information on Aging, #22*:1981, p. 3.

16. *Oxford English Dictionary,* Vol, II. Oxford, Claredon Press, 1933.

17. Wilensky, Harold L.: Work, careers, and social integration. *International Social Science Journal, 12*:554, 1960; the broader view of career such that it would include housewives, is held by Huges, Everett C.: Institutional office and the person. *American Journal of Sociology, 43*:441, 1937.

18. *Ibid.,* p. 554.

19. *Ibid.,* p. 555; Wilensky's quote from Mannheim, Karl: *Man and Society in an Age of Reconstruction,* Translated by E.A. Shils, New York, Harcourt, Brace, 1940, pp. 56, 104-106, 181.

20. Mannheim, Karl: *Essays in the Sociology of Knowledge.* New York, Oxford University Press, 1952, p. 248, cited by Cain, Leonard D., Jr., Life course and social structure. In Faris, Robert E.L. (Ed.): *Handbook of Modern Sociology,* Chicago, Rank McNally, 1964, p. 299.

21. Ariés, Phillippe: *Centuries of Childhood.* Translated by Robert Baldick, New York, Alfred A. Knopf, 1962, pp. 30-31.

22. Miller, D.C. and Form, W.: *Industrial Sociology: An Introduction to the Sociology of Work Relations.* New York, Harper, 1951, cited by Cain, Jr., Leonard D.: Life course and social structure, In Faris, Robert E.L. (Ed.): *Handbook of Modern Sociology.* Chicago, Rand McNally, 1964, p. 299.

23. Havinghurst, R.J.: The social competence of middle-aged people. *Genetic Psychology Monographs. 56*:297-375, 1957.

24. *Ibid.,* pp. 342-343.

25. William, Richard H.: Changing status, roles, and relationships. In Tibbitts, Clark (Ed.): *Handbook of Social Gerontology.* Chicago, University of Chicago Press, 1960, p. 288.

26. Von Mises, Ludwig: *Bureaucracy.* New Haven, Yale University Press, 1944, p. 97.

27. Reif, Fred and Strauss, Anselm: Rapid discovery and the scientific career. *Social Forces, 12*:297-311, 1965.

28. Glaser, Barney G.: Comparative failure in science. *Science, 143*:1012, 1964.

29. Scientists have been characterized as "idols oriented." *See* Eiduson, B.T.: *Scientists: Their Psychological World.* New York, Basic Books, 1962, p. 167.

30. For interesting speculation on the future relative to aging and meritocracy *see* Young, Michael: *The Rise of Meritocracy.* 1870-2033, London, Thames and Hudson, 1958, Chapter 4.

31. Haug, Marie R. and Sussman, Marvin S.: The second career — variant of a sociological concept. Read at the American Sociological Association Meeting, Miami, Sept. 1966, p. 5.

32. Wilensky, Harold L.: Orderly careers and social participation: The impact of work history on social integration in the middle mass. *American Sociological Review, 26*:525, 1961.

33. A work history of jobs that are functionally related and hierarchically ordered,

244   *The Social Consequences of Long Life*

but do not cross occupational strata could be defined as ordered within a lesser proportion of the work life. Wilensky uses one-fifth as the proportion.

34. Wilensky, *op. cit.*, p. 535.
35. For example, in the United States in 1890, 68.3% of all males over age 65 were in the labor force, whereas in 1970, the figure was 25.8%; U.S. Bureau of Census. *Statistical Abstract of the United States: 1971.* Washington, D.C., 1971, p. 211, and U.S. Bureau of Census, *Historical Statistics of the United States, Colonial Times to 1957.* Washington, D.C., 1960. p. 71.
36. Gorer, Geoffrey, An anthropologist considers retirement, In Gorer, G.: *The Dangers of Equality.* New York, Weybright & Talley, 1966, p. 151.
37. *Ibid.*, p. 152.
38. Thompson, Wayne E. and Streib, Gordon F.: Situational determinants: health and economic deprivation in retirement. *Journal of Social Issues, 14*:18-34, 1958; Tyhurst, J.S, Sald, L., and Kennedy, M.: Mortality, morbidity, and retirement. *American Journal of Public Health, 47*:1434-1444, 1957.
39. Back, Kurt W.: The ambiguity of retirement. In Busse, Ewald W. and Pfeiffer, Eric (Eds.), *Behavior and Adaptation in Late Life.* Boston, Little, Brown & Co., 1969, p. 10.
40. Orbach, Harold, L.: Normative aspects of retirement. In Tibbitts, Clark and Donahue, Wilma (Eds.): *Social and Psychological Aspects of Aging.* New York, Columbia University Press, 1962, p. 550.
41. Donahue, W., Orbach, H., and Pollak, O.: Retirement: The emerging social pattern. In Tibbitts, Clark (Ed.): *Handbook of Social Gerontology.* Chicago, University of Chicago Press, 1960, p. 382.
42. Streib, G.F. and Schneider, C.J.: *Retirement in American Society.* Ithaca, N.Y., Cornell University Press, 1971.
43. Tartler, Rudolf: The older person in family, community, and society. In Williams, R.H., Tibbitts, Clark, Donahue, Wilma, *et al., Processes of Aging.* New York, Atherton Press, 1963, p. 71.
44. *Ibid.*, p. 71.
45. Fried, Edrita G.: Attitudes of the older population groups toward activity and inactivity. *Journal of Gerontology, 4*:141-151, 1949.
46. Shanas, Ethel: The meaning of work, In Shanas, Ethel, *et al., Old People in Three Industrialized Societies.* New York, Atherton Press, 1968, p. 338.
47. Breen, Leonard Z.: Retirement — Norms, behaviors, and functional aspects of normative behavior. In Williams, Richard H., Tibbitts, Clark and Donahue, Wilma, *op. cit.*, p. 384.
48. Doyle, Jack: Green revolution II. New York *Times*, April 25, 1981, p. A23.
49. Lindsey, Robert: Older people hit hard by inflation are delaying retirement. The New York *Times*, August 17, 1980, p. 32; Special Report: Why many keep on job as long as possible. *U.S. News and World Report*, September 1, 1980, p. 58.
50. U.S. Department of Labor, *The Length of Working Life for Males.* 1900-1960, Manpower Report No. 8, Washington, Government Printing Office, July 1, 1963, p. 7-8.
51. Back, Kurt W.: The ambiguity of retirement. In Busse, Ewald W. and Pfeiffer,

Eric (Eds.): *Behavior and Adaptation in Late Life.* Boston, Little, Brown & Co., 1969, p. 100.
52. Donahue, W., Orbach, H., and Pollak, O.: Retirement: The emerging social pattern. In Tibbitts, Clark (Eds.): *Handbook of Social Gerontology.* Chicago, University of Chicago Press, 1960, p. 343.
53. Kreps, Juanita M.: Economics of retirement. In Busse and Pfeiffer: *op. cit.* p. 88.
54. *Ibid.*
55. The issue as defined does not face the fact that for those already retired, the only solution is to raise social security or otherwise provide greater retirement income, irrespective of previous work life earnings. *Ibid.,* p. 89.
56. *Ibid.,* p. 89.
57. *Ibid.,* p. 90-91.
58. Mayer, Kurt B.: Social stratification in two egalitarian societies: Australia and the United States. In Bendix, R. and Lipset, S.M. (Eds.): *Class, Status, and Power.* 2nd edition, New York, Free Press, 1966, p. 154.
59. Faltermayer, Edmund K.: The drift to early retirement. *Fortune,* May, 1965, pp. 113-114.
60. U.S. Department of Health and Human Services, Public Health Services, Vital Statistics of the United States, 1978, Vol. II, Section 5. *Life Tables,* Washington, D.C., U.S. Government Printing Office, 1980, pp. 5-13.
61. Rothenberg, Dan: Don't count on your pension. *Philadelphia Magazine,* 63, (December, 1972), p. 143.
62. The New York *Times,* Feb, 15, 1970.
63. *Ibid.*
64. Sarason, Seymour B.: *Work, Aging, and Social Change.* New York, The Free Press, 1977; Best, Fred: *Flexible Life Scheduling; Breaking the Education-Work-Retirement Lockstep.* New York, Praeger, 1980.
65. Laufer, Robert and Bengtson, Vern L.: Generations, aging, and social stratification: On the development of generational units. *Journal of Social Issues,* 30(3): 200, 1974.
66. Best, *op. cit.,* 1980, p. 73; Best referred to: Munnel, Alicia: *The Future of Social Security.* Washington, D.C., Brookings Institution, 1977, p. 79.
67. Sheppard, Harold L. and Rix, Sara E.: *The Graying of Working America: The Coming Crisis in Retirement-Age Policy.* New York, The Free Press, 1977, pp. 70-80.
68. This happened in some of the iron range communities in northern Minnesota.
69. Waring, Joan M.: Social replenishment and social change: The problem of disordered cohort flow. *American Behavioral Scientist,* 19(2):252, 1975.
70. *Ibid.,* p. 239.
71. *Ibid.,* p. 252.
72. *Ibid.,* p. 253.
73. *Ibid.,* pp. 253-254.

Chapter 10

LONG LIFE AND THE FUTURE

THROUGHOUT this book, an attempt has been made to point out and elaborate on some of the social consequences of long life. The changes that have taken place in the timing of death during the past two or three centuries have been considered important factors in shaping social life in modern society. By deliberately emphasizing the change in life expectancies, however, the danger of overemphasis is present.

Although the new phenomena relating to long life are important, its occurrence forms only one aspect of the many important changes that have appeared since the Industrial Revolution. I have tried to be mindful of Bennett Berger's warning: "the increasing numbers, decentralization, and specialization of intellectuals, the availability of print, the respectability of almost any scheme of values (as long as they are logically articulated), and our predilection to think that by naming something we understand it, all contribute to the helter-skelter rush with which we hasten to confer the status of 'trend,' 'movement,' 'spirit,' etc., on a series of events which, with some historical distance, we might recognize as a minor cultural quiver."[1] There seems little doubt that increased longevity is an established fact; the problem is determining the social meaning and consequences of that fact.

It is conceivable that the increased life expectancy over the entire life course may be considered comparable to such important developments as industrialization, advanced technology, population increase, urbanization, the rise of mass media, and mass education. The perspective needed to discern the meaning of changes in longevity may be a consequence of the future-oriented perspective discussed in Chapter 3. The mandatory role changes and the role choices that are open to long-lived affluent men and women require that they view their lives with a long-term perspective. This implies that they will recognize the relevance of history.

Marias states that Western man has only recently gained an "historical awareness."[2] Modern men and women have become conscious of the long sweep of history to a degree never before attained:

> We of the West have become increasingly aware of the fleeting, quickening pace of historical life and this very 'awareness' now functions as a new ingredient in our life and thus has become an additional factor in its acceleration. There is a difference between the actual acceleration of the historical tempo and men's knowing about it, just as there is between one's having a disease and knowing that one has it. It is no longer merely a question of considering an impression passively; it is a question of being alert to a change already foreseen and counted on — of anticipating the change.[3]

Historical awareness and a quickened tempo in contemporary events compel the individual to become self-conscious about the present and the future. Part of the impulse towards this kind of self-consciousness results from being alerted to a change already foreseen and counted on. That life is generally longer than ever before is one of the changes that has called forth new perspectives of what life might be under this circumstance.

Lifting the burden of imminent death and traditionalism lends itself to the shaping of new perspectives of the future as well as the past, as illustrated earlier by the Algerian peasant. The view of the past can only have utility for one who would use it as an aid to the explanation of the present and for building a theory or perspective that facilitates planning for the future. Since the development of memory, highly selected elements of the past have become part of human culture. It is only with the onset of circumstances that are conducive to self-conscious planning that the perspective of history thought important here could emerge. As stated, such a perspective has been affected by and contributed to the social consequences of long life.

It is possible that in earlier times and in places outside the influence of European society longevity was great enough to allow the emergence of life perspectives conducive to life course planning among ordinary men and women.

One of the questions arising from this discussion is how and when the demographic facts of life fully affect the social consciousness and contribute to the shaping of attitudes, values, and expectations; that is, under what conditions do long life expectancies result in social change. One might be tempted to assume that the actual experience of high or low death rates among family and age peers determine our perception of life expectancy. Vinovskis' work on death in colonial Massachusetts challenges such an assumption.[4] The early New Englanders put an extreme emphasis upon death every day of their lives, although their actual life expectancy was unusually long for the times. Death rates in New England in the seventeenth century were similar to those recorded in 1860, about 200 years later. Though many lived to advanced old age, they remained obsessed with the imminence of death and the specter of a short precarious life. These historical findings demonstrate that the relationship between demographic facts and social life are subtle and complex.

After studying death rates and related cultural phenomena of New England, Vinovskis concludes

> Perhaps now we are in a better position to account for the misconceptions of early New Englanders of the level of mortality in their society. They came from England where mortality rates were very high. Their expectations of continued high mortality in the New World were reinforced by the difficulties of the early years of settlement, the uncertainty of life due to the presence of periodic epidemics, and particularly high mortality of their children. Though their chances of survival in American were actually much better than those of their relatives and friends in the old country, they usually did not realize this fact because of the great emphasis that was placed on death by their religion. The continued reminder of the shortness of their lives whenever anyone died made it difficult for the average person to comprehend the changes in the overall mortality level that occurred.[5]

In addition to that, life in New England was lived on farms and in villages. When death occurs in a small intimate social setting even the death of a single individual can "leave a big hole."[6] Premature death in a society like New England meant that children might have to go to an orphanage or that a widow would be sent to the almshouse. There was no life insurance or Social Security. It is also apparent that throughout a large part of Colonial America, death rates were high and life was precarious. A short distance to the south of New England, in Delaware and Virginia, death rates from malaria were very high.

A set of findings similar to those found by Vinovskis in Massachusetts are reported in a study of the French working class at the turn of the century. Stearns found that most workers did not really expect to live to be old and their definition of old age in itself was distinctive. Both attitudes may have been passed down from rural tradition. High death rates, even though particularly among infants could create a disbelief in the likelihood of long life, even though the number of older villagers (like that of older workers later) was substantial. (Adult longevity, that is, life expectancy if one survived until 20, improved only about three years between 1780 and 1900.) . . . Debility among older villagers more probably formed the basis of the belief that the onset of old age was early. In both cases industrialization could easily enhance the traditional outlook. Continued high infant mortality, knowledge of older workers maimed and disabled (simply the loss of teeth by age 40 was dishearteningly visible), the tendency of old workers to disappear from view into other job categories or back to the countryside — all made it easy for a young worker to expect not to live even if statistically his chances of passing fifty-five were quite good.[7]

In the past, a great proportion of all death was premature, even by earlier standards of life expectancy. Premature deaths, according to Kurt Back, can be defined as crisis points: "In the study of the life course, the catastrophes correspond to the decision points, the events of life visible to the outsider. . . . Psychologically, we may call these crisis points, points where small imputs may lead to great change."[8]

When the timing of death changes and occurs more frequently at the older ages, life is relieved of a number of catastrophes or crises. That this is the case in modern societies at this time can be considered a measure of real progress.

Although the notion of human progress is questioned by many social scientists and philosophers, the history of the daily life in which we have gained control over some of the variables of "fate" referred to earlier seems to indicate that progress has occurred. This is particularly true if we take a long-term perspective and are sensitive to trends. Fourastié comments:

> No one seems to care at all about long term trends. No one seems to notice the passage of the popular masses from a vegetal life to one that is not so limited. Not a word is said about the disappearance of famines in the Western world. . . . No one seems to suspect the existence of factors favorable to individuality in the new tertiary civilization. A man who, two centuries ago, would not even have learned to read, if he had survived to maturity, profits by his windows, the central heating of his apartment, and the 300,000 copies of the newspaper for which he writes, to announce that humanity has arrived at the last stage of barbarism.[9]

Despite Fourastié's commentary one cannot help but be

discomfited by some of the major dilemmas of our time.

Long Life and Some Human Dilemmas

The social consequences of long life affect and are affected by a number of human dilemmas. Three of the most pervasive dilemmas resulting in conflict or tension are those between (a) rationality and spontaneity, (b) community solidarity and individuality, and (c) the desire for more freedom and the fear of or reluctance to take responsibility. Although these can be expressed separately, they are frequently interrelated to one another.

Longevity has in no way resolved the tension between rationality and spontaneity, although it may have increased the opportunity for both. For example, a future orientation requires rational planning on one hand and allows for spontaneity relatively free from dampening effects of great uncertainty and imminent death on the other.

The added time for living and its accompanying perspective have allowed for the late bloomer, while at the same time requiring rationality in the conduct of education and career planning. The time now allocated to childhood has not only provided a social place for the spontaneity of early years but has required rationality in education for full literacy, abstract thought, and scientific approach to knowledge. The increased allowable time for education, a result of high level productivity as well as the control of death, has put a premium on long-term plans and preparatory time. High level theoretical and technical training takes time, in fact most of one's time during the first twenty to twenty-five years of life.

A long period of education would seem conducive to rationality, especially if it is related to future life chances in employment and life-style. Time for the exercise of choice regarding training and career and a future-oriented perspective seem to tip the scales in favor of rationality. The direct rejection of rationality seen in the current popularity of astrology and the occult, for example, may be reactions to the exaggerated claims for the efficacy of rationality in the past.

The form of rationality made possible by longevity and the factors and circumstances related to it are associated with planning. As noted earlier, the prospect of having more than one career demands rational planning. The numbers able to engage in a lifetime that embraces more than one career is increasing with a resulting increase in rational decision-making.

The housewife whose children have been launched by the time she is forty can expect to live another thirty-five to forty years and will make a long series of choices, consciously or subconsciously. In pursuing a second career, the entry of women into the labor force is a rational act. Furthermore, the new postparental roles in the process of development, within the institution of the family, indicates the emergence of an added increment of rationality, at least until the postparental roles are fully institutionalized. To some, however, the middle-aged couples' postparental period of childlessness may appear fraught with irrationality. The increase in marital dissolution and resultant serial monogamy by choice rather than by death may be evidence of an increase in spontaneity.

Although it appears that long life has contributed to an increase in rationality, many social commentators have decried the lack of thought and rationality in contemporary life. Charles Fair writes, "As Alvin Toffler tells us, we live in an age of increasing pluralism — in tastes, in beliefs, in standards of morals and credibility."[10] Rather than stimulating judgement and thoughtful choice, Fair asserts that "far from thinking too much, the evidence is that we are thinking less and less — that our whole search is for ways to make ourselves sane and happy at the smallest possible cost in effort or responsibility."[11] Whether or not Fair is correct in his forecast of the demise of rationality and what he terms the "rational consensus" is uncertain. The resurgence of interest in fundamentalist religion, astrology, Tarot cards, and the occult may also be reactions against rationality and individual choice. The change in the timing of death may necessitate the self-conscious development of new institutional safeguards in the maintenance of rationality and freedom. Despite signs to the contrary, some aspects of rationality have increased.

Though longevity and the decline of uncertainty regarding death have contributed to spontaneity, long life seems to require added rationality. The rationality that goes into the planning necessary for those who spend a decade or more retired from active work did not have to be pursued in the past. The economic planning required in matters relating to investment in money market funds, retirement benefits, life insurance and part-time work after official retirement are all related to longevity. The family help patterns that are developing between parents and children within the middle levels of industrial society are also connected to long life. New norms of consumption involving the use of personal credit among the elderly require a degree of economic rationality that was unncessary when high rates of premature death made life more precarious.

As theories relating to health and long life have developed, a fatalistic orientation toward the anticipation of disability and death in late middle and old age seems to have decreased. The regimen required for health and the control of chronic diseases in old age assumes rational behavior. Living successfully with a chronic disease becomes a test of rationality.[12] A dilemma similar to that posed by the forces of rationality and spontaneity is that which emerges in the polarity between the desires of community on the one hand and individuality on the other.

Low infant mortality and the increases in life expectancy along the rest of the life course have meant a decline in community or social integration in the classical sense. Correspondingly, there has probably been an increase in individuality, although there is no exact inverse relationship between the degree of community solidarity and individuality. The shift from traditionalistic communal lifestyles to greater individual variation is partially the result of the great increase in population and the change away from the fatalism of traditional thoughtways.[13] The small, precariously based subsistence societies of the past could not tolerate a great deal of individuality. The rise of the large, highly productive occupationally diversified societies gave impetus to varied life-styles, anonymity, and social controls based upon legal standards and norms, all of which favor diversity and individuality. Modern circumstances have provided greater possibilities for choice, and choice is a major prerequisite for freedom and individuality.

The new conditions of life have helped create what Geiger refers to as two analytically distinct types of *social interdependence*. These emerge from the fact ". . . that people are dependent on one another for the maintenance of their physical existence, and second, that they have a psychological need for social intercourse with their own kind."[14] Geiger distinguishes these as *external* and *internal interdepen-*

dence.

> The first is manifested in orderly cooperation, the other in emotional community. External interdependence assumes the form of a united effort of a number of persons for the satisfaction of various kinds of needs. Internal interdependence manifests itself in sympathetic relationships between persons; one could almost say, as spiritual communion. The ego of the one is interwoven with the egos of others. He more or less identified himself with them, in extreme cases to the point of complete surrender of the self and total fusion. He cannot separate himself from the others or be torn from them without experiencing it as a kind of spiritual mutilation.[15]

In describing social evolution, Geiger states, "In societies with very primitive structures, one and the same social unit is held together by external as well as internal interdependence. Each accompanies, complements, and strengthens the other."[16] In advanced societies, the division of labor leads to specialization, and "the circle of active persons united in external interdependence becomes even greater. As standards of living rise, and demands for material goods and services increase, the range of interdependence includes not only economic activities, but develops on all levels of human activity and forms a "global culture."[17] "This social evolution, however, is accompanied by an individual one. With the development of his intellect, especially the capacity for abstraction and conceptual thinking, man changes from a herd-bound animal to an individual personality. The inner life of the individual gains independence, not in the sense that he retires from the community with others, but rather that he learns to distinguish between being-by-himself and being-with-others as two different modes of life and experience, between which he alternates according to situational circumstances."[18] The tension between individual and community make this a socially dynamic paradox.

The full recognition of the potentialities of long life can facilitate a more clearly defined approach to individuality in one instance and communal relations in the other. When more time can be spent in testing and judging the desirability of a particular life-style and vocational and avocational roles, the conditions exist for a more adequate resolution of this dilemma.

Much has been written lamenting the loss of community; the appeal for individuality is frequently given support in the same breath. Since neither aspect of human affairs can exist in pure form, life must contain elements of both. Some of the consequences of long life appear to increase the possibilities of functioning at both levels, and in this sense create a more adequate, multidimensional man. Nevertheless, modern life with wider choices and a forward-looking perspective is not likely to enhance the maintenance or development of the internal interdependence associated with full involvement in a life-long kin group, peer group, or work group; nor are these primary groups likely to be coextensive. However, modern men and women have the time and choice of circumstances to form various groups during a long life. In effect, as referred to earlier, the various periods of a long life will be lived with different kinds of social groups, and continuous relations with kinfolk, old friends, and acquaintances may cease to be functional. Old friends may not always be the best friends. New groups that are solid and intimate may be feasible and desirable as we develop the various sets of roles we must play in living out a long life. It is a life in which the social and biological circumstances change considerably throughout its course.

In responding to the need for a diverse number of secondary social relationships that are a part of the external interdependencies characteristic of modern life, Geiger further argues that we need to be more intellectualized, rather than pursue an emotional or sentimental approach to life. He claims that our traditional communal morality is too narrow. In opting for individuality over communality, Geiger emphasizes intellectuality:

> In modern society there is not so much a lack of "togetherness," but rather, in a certain sense, too much of it. The average person is not sufficiently capable of defending his inner interdependence against those social bodies which he is dependent on for his external existence. With all due reservations I wish to make a plea for the *emancipation of man from the community,* i.e., for his liberation from certain forms of emotional collectivism. It is not necessary to point out that an individualization in this sense goes hand in hand with intellectualization and is unthinkable without it. . . .[19]

The third dilemma is highlighted by the apparent contradiction of the desire for freedom on the one hand and the need for responsibility on the other. This dilemma is closely linked to the two already discussed. Both rationality and individuality would appear to enhance the potential for freedom, though it is a freedom conditioned by a complex of external interdependencies. A recognition of human interdependence brings the necessity for responsibility into sharp focus.

Long life and the relative diminution of the uncertainties of premature death have given new importance to freedom, while at the same time requiring the rationality inherent in planning ahead. The complexity of the structure of roles and the resulting interdependencies in modern society have enhanced the need for individual and collective responsibility. No longer can the conception of freedom without responsibility be tolerated on anything but a small scale. The prolongation of childhood and youthful dependence while being readied for adult life by education contributes to conceptions of freedom without responsibility. The denigration of middle and old age and the adulation of youth have also contributed to the dilemma.

Geographic mobility and short-term residence augment these modern dilemmas. Longevity makes long-term continuous residence in a single locality less functional than under circumstances of short life in which danger, disaster, and death were key features of the life course.

The precariousness of life before the nineteenth century curtailed the urge to move by families and individuals, with the exception of migration due to famine, pestilence, and war. Involvement in and dependence upon locality groups was so all inclusive that little time was spent in thinking about leaving kith and kin. If there was concern, it was probably in the fear that one would be forced to leave home and community.

With increased duration of life, changes in life-style impose the necessity of adapting to new age levels and environmental conditions. Frequently, it appears that part of the adaptation to change may be facilitated by changing one's habitat as one moves through the various ages of life. For example, many youths leave home for work or college and spend their lives away from their place of origin. A great many older Americans move to warmer climates.

Human beings are characterized by their ability to adapt. Longevity promotes attitudes and perceptions conducive to adaptation. Nevertheless, for real adaptation and change to occur, new roles appropriate to each of the later age levels must be institutionalized. As the new roles for older people emerge, a corresponding alteration of roles will take place among those at the younger levels, such as those in late middle age, middle age, adulthood, late youth, and finally in childhood. When the perspective and the roles are developed for a long and varied life, child-rearing practices will reflect the changes resulting from long life. The commonly held pattern of contemporary life, which calls for early marriage, an occupational niche, small family, retirement, and death, is too simple a model. This is especially true under conditions that permit individuals to have more than one occupational career, new friends, new wife or husband, new avocation, and new leisure time tastes all within a normal lifetime.

Life Expectancy in the Future

If we have left the impression that expected length of life will increase indefinitely, such is not the case. Although expected length of life has steadily increased for over two centuries, the human lifespan has probably remained at about a hundred years during the same period. Improved living conditions and more recently the biological and medical sciences have done a great deal to reduce our vulnerability to disease, but very little toward reducing the rate of aging. Furthermore, we are rapidly reaching the limits of longevity through the control of disease.

Robert Kohn states that the present limits to health and longevity are exemplified in Sweden: "The Swedish female population is one of the healthiest in the world; Swedish women enjoy the best health that can be attained in any culture. But this pattern of health, of life expectancy, has not changed substantially in about twenty years. This is but one sign of the end of progress in public health and vital statistics. By 1955, the limits of progress had been reached in terms of vital statistics, and nothing is going to change until we understand why the aging population is dying."[20] In the United States at present, 93 percent of newborn white females are expected to live to age fifty at least. Even if death among all of these females was eliminated before age fifty, the expected length of life at birth would only increase by five and one-half years.[21] Over half (three years) of this hypothesized five and one-half year gain would be achieved by preventing all deaths among those under twenty-five years of age.[22] Spengler states that decreasing this number much further can not be expected because there is a hard core of mortality among the younger age-groups. The aforementioned high, accidental death rates among seventeen- to eighteen-year-old American males, consititutes part of this problem.

The saving of some lives in infancy and youth may lead to premature deaths later on: ". . . If infant and child mortality is reduced to very low levels, individuals with hereditary defects survive into later years, usually to marry and perhaps pass on these defects to succeeding generations. Survival of less vigorous human strains, it is believed, may account in part for the failure of life expectancy at age sixty-five to increase significantly. Many of those who now escape infectious disease may be more prone to degenerative diseases than were those who did not die of infectious diseases in the past."[23] Within the next forty-five years, experts believe that disease controlling technologies will function so effectively that life expectancy at birth will increase to eighty-five years.[24] This will require almost full control over cardiovascular and cerebrovascular diseases and cancer.

Further advances in longevity will require the development of an explanation of the aging process. The emphasis must change from disease control to control over the rate of aging. That is, we will need to develop the means to extend the lifespan. This involves intervention in the aging process, which remains elusive. Our ability to unlock the secrets of aging in the near future are debatable. Experts who are looking into the future do not believe that the lifespan extending technologies will be available before 1990 or later, and that their effects will not be felt before the next century. Many of these techniques appear to be most effective if they are begun early in life. The technologies considered in future prolongation of the lifespan are grouped into four categories: "(1) Technologies that alter the cellular aging processes such as dietary control or supplementation; (2) Technologies that alter the aging of organ systems such as the reticuloendothelial system (resistance and immunity to infection); (3) Technologies that alter aging induced by organ systems such as hormone induced aging; (4) Tissue regeneration technologies."[25]

The Gerontological Society of America sent questionnaires to its members working in biological and medical fields. The question pertained to the prospects for increasing life expectancy after age sixty-five through the control of disease, control of rate of aging, or both by the year 2000. Thirty-four percent stated that they expected an increase of ten years (at the time, life expectancy at age sixty-five was fourteen years). An increase of five years was estimated by an additional 34 percent, and 20 percent estimated a two- to three-year increase. Twelve percent of the gerontologists believed life expectancy would remain the same, and 2 percent that it would decline.[26]

Although the gerontologists questioned are somewhat more optimistic than those who have given special study to the prospects for intervening in the aging process, a breakthrough in the biology of aging is yet to be made. Recent scientific history may indicate, however, that a conservative approach would be mistaken. "Only ten years ago, according to science writer Al Rosenfeld, many an emminent scientist rejected out of hand the possibility of recombining DNA. The same case can be made for the astounding rapidity with which microprocesses, microchips, and other microelectronics have effected the computer world; no one could have predicted it."[27]

Whether credence rests with the optimistic or conservative estimates of when further increases in life expectancy will occur, either viewpoint has policy implications for the technological countries of the world. One such policy concern is the great disparity between funding for research to control cardiovascular and cerebrovascular disease and cancer, and for gerontological research focused on the aging process. One hundred times more is currently spent on the former.[28] The cost effectiveness of the enormous expenditures needed to eliminate all cancer, for example, has been questioned. The increased length of life gained from the elimination of all cancer is 2.3 years at birth and 1.2 years at age sixty-five.[29] Some gerontologists believe that a shift of funds toward greater research efforts in explaining or merely slowing the aging process might yield more progress toward longer life, greater vigor, and fewer disabilities among the elderly. Moreover, the prevention or control of all cancer is not enough to push the expected length of life at birth to eighty years.[30]

Whether or not the control of heart disease, stroke, and cancer add a great deal to life expectancy is not as important as the effect such a development would have on life perspective and the social consciousness. Though we have a relatively long life expectancy if we live beyond infancy, we are almost inevitably faced with considerable apprehension about cancer and heart disease in middle and old age. The subtle apprehension felt by many people results from the uncertainty surrounding these diseases. For example, we often do not suspect that we have contracted one of these diseases until it is too late for treatment. Much of the current fadism in health foods and exercise regimens express the underlying hope that the right food and exercise will spare us from heart disease or cancer.

The control of these diseases could have a powerful effect on the life perspective of the middle-aged and older population; our perception of the aging process would be changed. Also, if we consider the prospect of the future control of arthritis and rheumatism, much of the negative connotation of aging might be sharply curtailed.

Reducing the apprehension of premature death and suffering from these degenerative diseases could eliminate much of the fear-inspired planning and activity of middle age. Present-day apprehension among the middle aged in the middle class stimulates the acceleration of plans for travel and other activities that would be impossible if one of these diseases attacked. When concerns of this type result in a panic to get valued things done in a race against time, the prospect of advancing age takes on a negative cast.

Greater control of the debilitating diseases of old age would provide more predictability in approaching old age. The conception that one ought to complete certain highly valued activities by age fifty-five to sixty would be changed if the fears regarding the relationship between age and disease were altered. Greater predictability would allow and encourage future plans that would reach into the seventy's and early eighty's. The realization that one could rationally plan and have choices between alternative activities and life-styles would reduce the apprehensions of approaching old age. Present-day uncertainty regarding the future does much to cause middle age malaise, midlife crisis, and deliberate avoidance of thinking about old age.

Decreasing the imminence of death for a decade or more after age sixty-five would have a decided effect on the future orientation of those in the last phase of the life course. Currently, most people over sixty-five years feel that they have a present and a past, but little or no future.

Freedom from imminent death until the end of the lifespan death at ages ninety to a hundred would not eliminate all the problems associated with individual responses to longevity. With a continuation of rapid social and cultural change, increases in life expectancy might result in creating individuals who are destined to "live through a succession of societies in the course of a life time."[31] At present, we are not prepared for such a change in the later part of the life course. "The life projects we had for a much more circumscribed life expectancy will no longer be adequate for longer life expectancy."[32] Nevertheless, the new mortality schedules and changes in life perspective will encourage us to develop adequate life projects in the future.

Present-day policy planners view the economic problems of longevity as most important. Their concern is aptly illustrated by the following quotation: "Although the elderly represent only 10 percent of the population, they —

Use 29 percent of the total cost of health care.
Make 60 percent more physician visits than the middle aged.
Occupy at least 30 percent of acute hospital beds.
Receive 25 percent of the total number of prescriptions.
Occupy 95 percent of the nursing home beds.
Utilize 20 percent of physician office time."[33]

In addition to this, the Department of Health and Welfare estimated that between 1978 and 2025 the cost of Medicare and Medicaid for those over sixty-five will increase ten fold.[34] Preston has calculated that if we eliminate cardiovascular disease and cancer within the next thirty years, the proportion of population over age sixty-five would increase by 74 percent. If, in turn, we wished to maintain the present proportion between active workers and retirees in the United States, we would have to postpone the average retirement age by approximately twelve years.[35]

The change in timing of the major events of aging may improve the aging process. Nevertheless, there is little evidence that the projected increases in expected length of life at the older ages will allow the very old to escape a period of preterminal deterioration, although the length of this period might be relatively short.

The social changes accompanying present and future increases in longevity imply that serious measures need to be taken to prepare present and future populations. Kaplan states "It will require intensive educational orientation both formal and informal at all levels of schooling to change cultural views about old age held by the old as well as others. It will necessitate the introduction of content about aging into our elementary schools through the higher educational system which trains teachers."[36]

The consequences of the increase in life expectancies are being felt in modern societies. Longevity has, however, yet to affect the lives of people in the developing countries of the world. For them, the next half century will be a period of transition from a death ridden past to a prolonged and more stable life course in the future. The response to a new chronology of life and death will vary considerably. Differences in culture will dictate the degree of change and the nature of consequences. The younger cohorts that experience the social, psychological, political, and economic impact of new ways of living the life course will be profoundly affected. The new attitudes, values, and expectations associated with changes in the timing of death, potentialities of a long lifetime, and new definitions of aging are fundamental. The resultant changes may be revolutionary.

REFERENCES AND NOTES

1. Berger, B.M.: How long is a generation. *British Journal of Sociology, 11*:19, 1960.
2. Marias, J.: *Generation: A Historical Method.* Translated by Raley, H.C.: University, Alabama, University of Alabama Press, p. 7.
3. *Ibid.,* p. 9.
4. Vinovskis, M.A.: Angels heads and weeping willows: death in early America. In Hareven, T.K. (Ed.): *Themes in the History of the Family.* Worcester, American Antiquarian Society, 1978, pp. 39ff.
5. *Ibid.,* p. 53-54.
6. Blauner, R.: Death and social structure. *Psychiatry, 29*:378-94, 1966.
7. Stearns, P.N.: Aging in the working class: an exploratory essay. *International Labor and Working Class History,* No. *8,* Nov. 1975, p. 22.
8. Back, K.: Mathematics and the poetry of human life and points in-between. In Back, K.W. (Ed.): *Life Course: Integrative Theories and Exemplary Populations.* Washington, D.C., AAAS, 1980, p. 167.
9. Fourastié, J.: *The Causes of Wealth.* New York, Free Press, 1960, p. 229.
10. Fair, C.: *The New Nonsense: End of the Rational Consensus.* New York.
11. *Ibid.*
12. The number of people suffering chronic diseases has increased markedly in recent decades, a fact that is clearly related to the increase in the aged population.
13. Notwithstanding the recent interest in communes in the U.S.
14. Geiger, T.: *On Social Order and Mass Society: Selected Papers.* Edited by Mayntz, R., translated by Peck, R.E. Chicago, University of Chicago Press, 1969, p. 222; Geiger's internal and external interdependence is very similar to the dichotomies of Durkheim (mechanical and organic solidarity), Maine (custom and contrast), Tönnies (gemeinschaft and gesellschaft), and Weber (traditional

and legal order).

15. *Ibid.*, p. 223.
16. *Ibid.*, p. 223.
17. *Ibid.*, p. 223.
18. *Ibid.*, p. 223.
19. *Ibid.*, p. 187-88.
20. Kohn, R.: Biomedical aspects of aging. In Van Tassel, D.D.: *Aging, Death and the Completion of Being.* Philadelphia, Pa., University of Pa. 1979, p. 4.
21. Spengler, J.J.: *Population and America's Future.* San Francisco, W.H. Freeman, 1975, p. 8.
22. *Ibid.*, p. 8.
23. *Ibid.*, p. 9.
24. Select Committee on Aging. U.S. House of Representatives, 96th Congress. Report of the Subcommittee on Human Services: *Future Directions for Aging Policy: A Human Service Model.* Washington, D.C., 1980, p. 110; The information reported came from: Gordon, T.J., Gerjnoy, H. and Anderson, M.: *A Study of Life Extending Technologies.* Glastonbury, Conn., The Futures Group, Nov. 1977.
25. *Ibid.*, p. 112.
26. Neugarten, B.L. and Havighurst, R.J. (Eds.): *Extending the Human Life Span: Social Policy and Social Ethics.* Chicago, Committee on Human Development, University of Chicago, 1977, p. 51.
27. Select Committee on Aging, *op. cit.*, p. 112.
28. *Ibid.*, p. 103.
29. *Ibid.*, p. 102.
30. Keyfitz, N.: Improving life expectancy: an uphill road ahead. *Am J. of Pub. Health, 68(10)*:956, 1978.
31. Neugarten, *op. cit.*, p. 56.
32. *Ibid.*, p. 53.
33. Select Committee on Aging, *op. cit.*, p. 105.
34. *Ibid.*, p. 105.
35. Preston, S.H.: *Mortality Patterns in National Populations: With Special Reference to Recorded Causes of Death.* New York, Academic, 1976, p. 185.
36. Kaplan, J.: The effect of the extension of life on undergraduate academic gerontology. In Meltzer, M.M., Sterns, H., and Hickey, T. (Eds.): *Gerontology in Higher Education: Perspectives and Issues.* Belmont Ca., Wadworth, 1978, p. 93.

NAME INDEX

SUBJECT INDEX

A

Achievement and future orientation (*see* future orientation)
Achievement potential, 206
Adrenalin, 36
Adulation of youth, 90
Age
 and diversity, 117
 and feminine "attractiveness," 136
 and individualism, 111
 and loss of status, 114
 and normlessness, 114
 and obsolescence, 172
 and role loss, 114-118
 and use of status symbols, 186-189
Age composition
 change in, 214
Age Discrimination Act, 233
Age-grade
 lock step system of, 166
Age-grading, 115
Age-grading system, 167
Ageism in American society, 205
Age of science, 162
Age relevant society, 86
Ages of life, 6
Aging and embarrassment, 81-82
Aging establishment, 99
Aging and failure, 81-82
Aging and leisure, 118-121
Alcoholic problems, 94
Alexander the Great, 195
Alienation of eldely, 111
American colonial towns, 19
American Council on Life Insurance, 160
American families
 economic strength of, 155
American farmers, 61, 62
American high school, 54
American life, 146
American males, accidental deaths of, 257

American Revolution, 58
American schools, 164
American Way of Life, 58
American workers, 118
American youth, 71
Amicable Society for a Perpetual Assurance, 153
Algerian peasants, 44, 54, 56, 57, 60, 64, 247
Annual duration of work, 211
Anomie, 141
Anopheles mosquito, 36
Anticipatory socialization, 146
Anti-heros, 122
Area Redevelopment Act, 172
Arizona, 117, 235
Army Alpha test, 173
Arteriosclerosis, 91
Arthritis and rheumatism, 91, 123, 259
Ascensionism, 58
Asiatic cholera, 25
Assistant Secretary of Labor, 234
Aureomycin®, 36

B

Bacteriology, 36
Battle of Hastings, 21
Bengal, 25
Beriberi, 31
Bills of Mortality, 153
Birth cohorts, 4, 13, 14, 37, 75, 76, 84, 89, 107, 115, 144, 150, 161, 174
Birth control, 60
Birth defects, 22
Black Death, 17, 22, 23, 24, 50, 180
Blasphemies against God, 50
Body preoccupation, 90
Body transcendence, 90
Boredom, 52, 83, 93, 94
Breslau, 1687-1691, 15, 153
British Isles, 27
British Poor Inquiry Commission, 29

Functional disorders, 95
Future orientation
 and achievement, 57-65
 and individuality, 65
 and longevity, 54-57

G

Gastrointestinal parasitosis, 31
General Board of Health, 35
Generation gap, 150, 209
Genetic aspects of disease, 123
Genetic engineering, 123
Geneva, 26
Genoa, Italy, 25
Genocide, 72
Geographic mobility, 184
Geriatric care, 13
Geriatric medicine, 94
Geriatrics, 5, 13, 124
German concentration camps, 50
Germany, 107
Gerontological Society of America, 257, 258
Gerontology, 5, 89, 94, 104, 117, 124, 189, 194
Global culture, 253
God's Law, 183
God's wrath, 24
Grandparenthood, 141ff
Great Britain, 27, 107
Greek mythology, 58
Green revolution, 230
Greystoke, England, 28
Guaranteed minimum incomes, 62

H

Hamburg, Germany, 23
Hamlet, 17
Hard core poor, 64
Harvard College, 162
Health life expectancy, 237
Heart disease, 91, 123, 125
Henry, VIII, 12
Heroic models (Romantic), 122
H.E.W. data, 237
High and low energy societies, 109
Hippie life-style, 170
Hippie phenomenon, 122
Hiroshima, 50

Historical awareness, 247
Holland, 110
Horatio Alger myth, 58
Hospice, 125
Human genetics, 13
Hungary, 21
Hundred Years War, 24

I

Ideology of individuality, 153
Illness
 escape and, 121
 deviant behavior and, 121
Impaired hearing, 92
Income curve, 185
India, 27, 37, 38
Indian cholera (*see* Asiatic cholora)
Individuality and future orientation (*see* Future orientation)
Indo-China war, 47
Indonesians, 54
Industrial revolution, vii, 19, 23, 29, 57, 162, 198, 246
Industrialization and status of the elderly, 198
Infant death rates, 140
Infant mortality, 5, 48, 69, 138
Infant mortality rates
 control of, 149
 decline of, 149
Infectious disease, 13, 51, 70, 123
Inheritance, long life and, 191-193
Insulin, 36
Insurance
 long life and, 152-156
 medical, 98
Intergenerational mobility, 185
Intimacy, 82, 83, 84
I.Q., 613
 decrease in, 174
 research in, 173
Ireland, 28, 29, 42
Isolation, 93
Italy, 109

J

Japan, 230

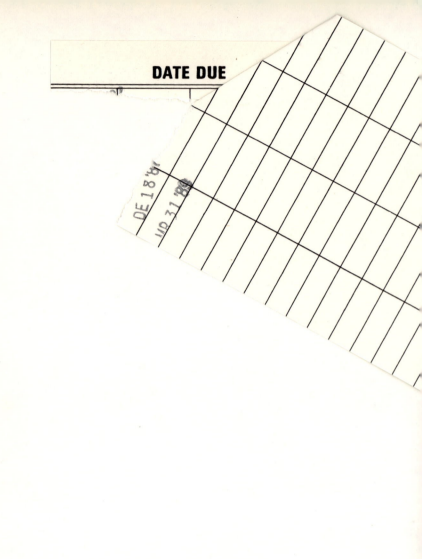

DATE DUE

DE 18 '84

JJD 31 '86